Sarah Boston is a documentary film maker and writer. Her books include *A History of Women Workers and The Trade Unions*, *Disorderly Breasts*, *Merely Mortal* (which accompanied a Channel 4 documentary series) and the award winning *Will, My Son*. She was born in Zimbabwe, spent her childhood in Yorkshire and now lives in London.

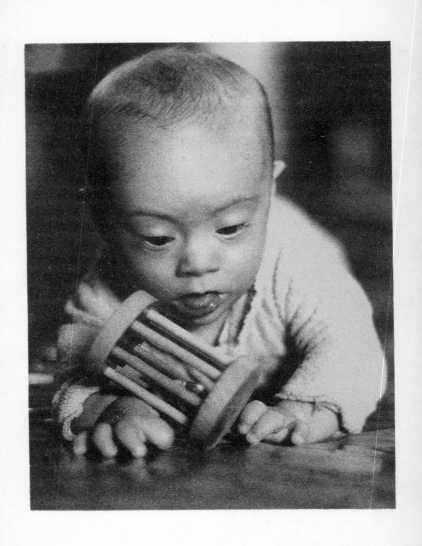

Sarah Boston

TOO DEEP
FOR TEARS

*Eighteen years after
the death of Will, my son*

Pandora
An Imprint of HarperCollinsPublishers

Pandora
An Imprint of HarperCollins*Publishers*
77-85 Fulham Palace Road,
Hammersmith, London W6 8JB
1160 Battery Street,
San Francisco, California 94111-1213

First published by Pandora, 1994

10   9   8   7   6   5   4   3   2   1

A catalogue record for this book
is available from the British Library

ISBN 0 04 440891 9

Typeset by Harper Phototypesetters Limited,
Northampton, England
Printed in Great Britain

For Ed

Contents

He weighed 4 lb 6 oz at birth and 14 lb 6 oz at death. He spent 34 weeks in the womb and should have stayed there 40 weeks. He lived for 40 weeks. He should have had 46 chromosomes in each cell but he had 47. He was born on 14 February, St Valentine's Day and died on 20 November. His heart failed him. He was called Will. He was my son.

The bald facts of the brief life of a mentally handicapped child with a severe congenital heart defect might sound to some like a tragic aberration in the normal cycle of human reproduction. As such they regard it as best ended and hopefully forgotten. To me the nine months of his life was an affirmation of life. As such it could never be 'best ended' and should not be forgotten.

Will, My Son, 1981

Will has not been forgotten. At each anniversary of his birth I remember him and wonder what might have been. Since his death, I have lived both with the memory of him and with the person that I am because of his life and death. Part of me died when he died, but the rest of me that survived has been immeasurably enriched by the brief life of my son, Will.

I live with my personal loss but we, as a society, face a collective loss as those who regard such lives as a 'tragic aberration in the normal cycle of human reproduction' are in the ascendancy. People with Down's Syndrome enrich our society and our understanding of what it is to be human. Their lives, like Will's life, are an affirmation of life. 'They' cannot be 'best ended'.

Too Deep For Tears, 1994

Introduction

WILL, MY SON

> I remember Will mostly in calm, but sometimes even now memories jog me and I break. I still want to talk about him not so much because I any longer have a need but because to be silent about him is to deny his existence.

These two sentences began the final paragraph of *Will, My Son* (Pluto Press, 1981). The first sentence holds as true now as it did then. The second sentence held true only, I now know with hindsight, for that moment in time. Finishing the book gave me a sense of being talked out. Little did I realize then that this feeling was but a pause in the conversation. My need to talk about him continued and continues still. *Will, My Son* was a very public way of speaking out and ensuring that his existence was not denied. Its publication also plunged me into a new relationship – a relationship with others through a third party, my book.

Books, once published, have a life of their own. Before the publication of *Will, My Son* I was apprehensive of the possible emotional repercussions of going public with such a personal story. What I had not anticipated was that the book, as a separate entity from me, would influence my life, my relationships and the lives of others. I have written other books, before and after *Will, My Son* but my relationship to them is quite different. It is more professional, much less personal. Their conception, even though based on my ideas, was also much more professional. When I started to write *Will, My Son*, the initial impetus was purely personal.

I wrote *Will, My Son* out of necessity. I felt compelled to try to transfer experiences, feelings and emotions that continually replayed in my head on to paper. I did not even think about the possibility of publishing it. Later I was to find out that this compulsion to write is shared by many who have been bereaved. For me, there was a desperate need to try to find some mental calm, and it was this that spurred me to write. I had been through four years of emotional turbulence, during which I had been frightened to pause for reflection. I wrote of the year following Will's death that:

> Behind everything I did there was a driving force - the fear of stopping. I felt I had to keep running because to stop was to think and to think was to remember. I hadn't come to terms with Will's death. My grief remained close to the surface. My life was one largely of evasion, my actions motivated by reaction to Will's death.

In fact, I kept running for four years. Running through the pregnancy and birth and first two years of life of my second child, Jessie. It was only when I had reached a degree of emotional safety, helped by a sense of security that Jessie was normal and healthy, that I could pause to think. To think was still to remember. After four years, writing was, for me, like booking myself on to an intensive course of therapy. What, in my ignorance, I did not realize was that I would, over the years and in different ways, have to book myself in for further sessions. Grief, I have learned, is for life.

The first draft of this then untitled book was written very intensively and quickly. When I had finished, I read and reread it and, in so doing, began to wonder if others might be interested in my experiences and find them of some use. During this period, my urge 'to say something' more public about the wider social, ethical and medical issues surrounding the birth and death of a Down's Syndrome child grew stronger. Finally, very tentatively, I gave the manuscript to a few people whose judgement I thought I would value. I misjudged one of them, or rather, he misjudged the manuscript. I had given it to him because he is someone with an honourable track record in broadcasting and the concerns of the disabled. His response to the manuscript was negative. He advised me to put it away and forget about it. It was, in his view, both too personal and too political. The content clearly embarrassed him and he was unable to talk about it in any way. Fortunately, the others were positive in their response and encouraged me to pursue publication.

I redrafted the book, acting on some of the advice and comments the other 'readers' had made. I then gave the manuscript to my partner, Ed to read. As my partner and the father of Will, his agreement was a precondition for my seeking a publisher. It was a long time before he read it. As someone who devours print, I knew that shortage of time was not the reason for his procrastination. I was deeply hurt by his apparent lack of interest and, yet, I knew that what stopped him was not lack of interest, but fear. Fear of what I might have written about him, fear of the pain and grief it might trigger, fear of thinking that what I had written was no good and having to tell me. Finally, he did read it, and his relief was visible. Although apprehensive about our personal life being made public, he fully supported my search for a publisher.

The next step was to send the manuscript out, through my agent, to publishers and test the response. Two or three turned it down, including one feminist press. This particular publisher was about to publish a novel in which the pain of a couple who give their Down's Syndrome baby to others to care for was explored. It seemed that, in some way, *this* was felt to be the feminist option, whereas my story of our decision to keep Will was somehow reactionary. I found this implied judgement deeply hurtful and confusing. With devastating irony, the rejection from another publisher was based primarily on what they felt was an unacceptable intrusion of feminism into the story! In an act of extraordinary insensitivity, this publisher passed on to me the readers' reports. Reading them was devastating.

The passages in *Will, My Son* that triggered the most extreme personal criticism by these readers were related to my admission of feelings, while pregnant, of ambivalence about and fears of having a child. Of the problem facing women in general I wrote, 'For any woman it is almost impossible to know before having a first child how it will affect them and their lives.' This concern, in relation to myself, I put in more forceful terms.

Despite my forward planning I still feared the worst. I not only feared that having a baby would at best interrupt and at worst end all that I had worked towards, I also feared the many other ways it might affect my life. When I was about five months' pregnant I wrote the following in a diary which rather dramatically sums up what my fears were: 'Everything I value will come to an abrupt halt in that tearing, searing, bloody moment of birth. I will no longer be a free agent. Another person's life will be utterly dependent on me. It will take my flesh, my blood, my life and there is no escape. My job opportunities will be severely restricted, my privacy invaded, my time taken and my youth. I fear the effect it will have on my relationship with Ed. I fear the effect it will have on me. I fear for the child I have conceived, my ego trip, whose life is already being moulded inside me.'

The thrust of these readers' criticisms, and, in one case, outright hostility and attacks on my personality, centred on the politics. For all of these critics, my 'feminism' was the heart of the problem. It not only led to what they viewed as the intrusion of unnecessary autobiographical material, but, also, to an unacceptable critique of the medical profession.

Not surprisingly, I found the personal nature of the criticisms deeply hurtful, but the political undercurrent of the attack spurred me on to seek a publisher. If this modest book, written not primarily with any political motive, could so threaten established attitudes, then its message clearly had importance. Soon after receiving this rejection, Stuart Hood, who had been a supporter of my manuscript from the outset recommended it to Pluto Press. They read it, responded positively and the processes of publication were put into motion.

The politics of the book were attractive to Pluto, but the personal, autobiographical aspect made them uneasy. Their unease was more in terms of the marketability of the product than their own response to it. *Will, My Son* is simply, as the subtitle explains, an account of *The Life and Death of a Mongol Child*. For me it was a book about a personal experience that changed me at the profoundest level. Because I am a feminist and have political views, they imbued my reactions to the experience, and it was natural for me to include them. For the publisher, however, my book did not fall into any set category.

Finally, it was listed as Autobiography/Social Studies/Health. Human experience does not fit neatly into categories. However, despite Pluto's unease about trying to market this hybrid book, they took the plunge. Apart from tidying up my grammar and punctuation, Pluto did not in any way change or try to change my text. I was particularly pleased that Pluto were very responsive to my suggestions for a cover design. I felt very strongly that there should be a photograph of Will either in the book or on the front cover. This was to show him as he was – a human being. It was to counter imagery born of ignorance. It was to counter the kind of image I had had when I was told that my ten-day-old son was Down's Syndrome, which was of 'a child with an abnormally large head, the slanted eyes associated with mongolism and a vacant face'. I had learned just how wrong my image was, and I wanted others to learn, too. Seeing someone with learning difficulties as a person, not as an image created as a result of ignorance, is to take the first step in acceptance.

From the very few photographs we had of Will, we selected two. On the front of the book is a picture of him lying on his stomach, concentrating hard on a wooden rattle he has in his hands. On the back, there is a picture of him, in my arms, gazing up into my eyes and we are smiling at each other. In both photographs, there is nothing vacant about his face. I wanted this strong imagery of his humanity to inform the reader when I talked about Down's Syndrome, mental handicap and abnormality. Once the book was published, many people commented on the photos. The most eloquent description of the effect of the photos was in a review of the book for the *Evening Standard* by Bel Mooney. She wrote, 'On the cover of the book are two photographs: in one a child who could have been written off is smiling up at his mother; in the other he struggles after a little wooden toy, fixed for ever in his striving by the click of the shutter. It is impossible not to be moved by that effort; impossible not to feel that you know him as a person – and that knowledge is the first step towards real compassion. There is no question about Will's importance. He will live forever – a smiling mongol baby – in the imaginations of all who read the book, reminding us of our most grave and joyful duty to respect life and give love'.

As publication date approached, I felt fear rising in me, a fear approaching terror. My terror was centred on my knowledge that Will, for me, lived on in the book. The book was much more than a way of speaking against a silent denial of his existence; it was a way of creating immortality for him. As an atheist, I do not believe in an afterlife. Much as I would, at times, have liked to have believed that he lived on some place else, I could never make such a leap of imagination, but, writing *did* keep him alive. Publication of the story of his life in book form meant that my son, thus immortalized, would go out into the world. In this process, then, for me, 'The word was made flesh' and, like any mother, I was terrified of how the world would respond to my son.

One of the elements of my fear, which was based on the readers' reports, never materialized. I expected some savage criticism, but it never came. For a modest publication from a small publisher, the book was widely reviewed. This was due largely to the generosity of my friend, Veronyka Bodnarec, who, having read the manuscript, offered to do the publicity free of charge. All the reviews were good, none attacked my feminism and the only hint of criticism crept in from one or two reviewers who felt that I was a little critical of the medical profession.

The culmination of the good public response was being informed that *Will, My Son* had won one of The Independent Order of Odd Fellows' Social Concern Awards.

The competition had been stiff that year, for 1981, the year of its publication, was the International Year For The Disabled. A plethora of books on the subject of disability had been published and submitted to the Order of Odd Fellows for consideration. It was, with huge pride, therefore, that I went up to receive the award at a reception at the House of Lords. For the audience, I was a winning author receiving a prize, but inside I knew that, first and foremost, I was a proud mother in a new dress (the most expensive dress I have ever bought), accepting an award on behalf of my son, for it was his particular quality, which lived on in the book, that touched people. It was only after this that I felt the award was for me, the author.

The very first responses of friends who read the book made it clear that their perception of me had changed, however slightly, as a result. Putting the experience on paper made people, even those who knew us closely, realize in graphic detail exactly what we had been through. It left them with a sense of awe that I recognized from my own experience.

The first time I had felt awe when confronted directly by another's pain was after the death of my elder sister's first child, Sarah. Immediately after her daughter's death, my sister, Louise, had gone to my parent's house. As soon as I got the news, I went there, too. That first night I slept with her. I remember lying in bed next to her and feeling in total awe of her. Her experience was beyond my imagination, her pain beyond my comprehension, and yet I felt the unspeakable depth of this pain.

For most people, the death of a child is their worst fear. One is left at a distance to wonder at the survivors of such experiences. This distance leaves one speechless. Many simply couldn't speak to me about my experiences, either at the time or after reading my book. The most that was said to me by those who read the book was that they had found it very moving. Although I had written about my experiences and, thus, was signalling that I was prepared to make my feelings public, most people eschewed talking to me about them. Social embarrassment surrounded the whole subject, and still does.

I was delighted that my friends read the book. To me, their act of reading it was confirmation of their support and understanding. The fact that they had not necessarily appreciated at the time what we were going through was not because of their lack of interest. My need to talk was much greater afterwards than while Will was living. So much of the nine months of his life was taken up with the all-consuming activity of looking after a small baby as well as dealing with the major traumas. To survive physically and psychologically, I had to just keep going and believe in a future for him. Doing, not talking, was one of my ways of coping at that time.

For those who had known me through the experience, the fact that I knew they knew was enough. The problem, over the years, has been with new friends or new potential friendships. At some point in a developing friendship, or even a close work collaboration, you explore each other's past. Chatting about parents, siblings, schooling, love affairs, children, politics and past experiences is all part of building up mutual understanding and friendship. In this process, you find differences and similarities, points of contact and of conflict. Some of your past is contained in the present. My 16-year-old daughter, Jessie, and my 23-year relationship with Ed are past *and* present and, therefore, obviously part of me and my life. Will, in terms of all outward evidence, is part of my past. I, therefore can choose to speak of him or not.

In fact, I feel I have *no* choice in this as, at some point in a developing friendship, I feel that it is very important for me to communicate that the person I am at present is informed by the experience of Will's life and death. Most register the information and some have followed up their interest by reading my book. I do not need them to comment or talk about the book. I am not looking for praise or to establish my credentials, as I might when showing someone a documentary film I have directed. I just need to know that they know. There are two levels for me when communicating this part of my history. One is the short version – a sentence that briefly relates that I had a Down's Syndrome son who died. This version, however, does not begin to touch on the depth of the experience. To tell the longer version is difficult and giving my book to someone to read is the easiest, least painful way I have found of enabling them to be aware of my past. For me to feel at ease in the friendship, I have to feel that my past is open and not some embarrassing, half-mentioned secret. I have to be able to talk of Will if and when I feel it is appropriate.

A few times, I have found a non-response to my past and to my book. What has thrown me about the non-response has been my misjudgement of the person concerned. Of course, lots of people I meet I would not expect to read my book and it is of no importance to me whether or not they do. However, on a very few occasions, I have wanted a person to read my book and have even gone as far as to give them a copy. Once I gave the copy to a film director acclaimed for his dramatic and sensitive 'fictional' films exploring his own childhood. He lost the copy and thought he might have left it on a plane. It was clear that this was a subject he simply couldn't deal with. Like one of my first 'readers', he was embarrassed by the direct, autobiographical nature of the story and would have been hugely more comfortable if it had been fictionalized.

Rather simplistically, I wrote off this and the earlier experience with my 'readers' as being the inability of most men to deal with feelings, with real human experience, with life and death. My mistake was to think that these two, because of their professional work, were different. Another mistake was to assume that women, because they are women, can deal with the book. Of course, there have been exceptions to this assumption. I have been close to women who carry their own grief and I know that reading my book would trigger too much pain for them, but some other women friends I blindly assumed would or could read it. I found out that some could not. They too, for their own reasons, find the subject too uncomfortable and are unable to even begin to look at it.

In general, though, my experience is that far more women have read the book than men, and I suspect that if a readership survey were to be carried out, this would be confirmed. Part of the female readership would be accounted for by those professionals, mainly women (nurses, midwives, health visitors and so on) who read it as part of their studies, but there is more to it than this. It is not just that women are more open to the content, they are more accepting of the style.

When I wrote *Will, My Son* it never occurred to me that there was anything odd about the style. The slip from the personal to the political, from describing an experience to making comment about the wider issues, merely reflected the flow of my life and thought. This interweaving of the different aspects of life comes naturally to most women. My experience of working with women is that the conversation can move from periods to polemics and back again in a seamless flow. For most men, life, and their conversations, are much more neatly divided. After Will's death and the immediate period of mourning, I took refuge in this division and explained my reasons for doing so.

I chose my main form of doing, 'work', for a variety of reasons. It was helpful to me not just because I found it interesting and absorbing. It was a refuge too. The world of work is well protected from the world of babies, children and motherhood. The separation of society into self-contained worlds, particularly the separation between work and children and the home is one I deplore, a separation that is a product of an industrialized, male-dominated society. Because of the respective roles of men and women it is a separation which most men have not questioned, but many women have. A working mother cannot help but be aware that her life cannot be so neatly and conveniently divided. Fortunately more and more people, both men and women, are becoming aware of those divisions and are questioning them but radical change seems a long way off. Much as I deplore it, I took advantage of it for that period of my life. As a childless woman I could take refuge in that separation.

It was a phoney refuge. Emotionally I could not make this separation and as a human being, I did not want to make it. It was natural, then, that when I came to write, I would interweave the various parts of my life. I found that I had written a book that did not fit into the neat divisions of the publishing market. The interweaving threatened these divisions and, implicitly, threatened the way most men organize their minds, emotions and lives. It was hardly surprising that most women found the style of *Will, My Son* as seamless as their conversations, but men could not get into it.

I only became aware of the threatening nature of the style of the book some years later when I delivered a manuscript about breast cancer to a publisher. The editor assigned the manuscript set about rewriting it. The content he accepted, but he had strong ideas about the style. He felt that the everyday, non-medical language and the personal approach to the subject was inappropriate. Making very heavy weather of it, he started a major, stylistic rewrite. Fortunately for me, in the middle of this battle of the rewrite, the publishing company went into liquidation and another publisher, headed by a woman, took on the manuscript. She read it and positively liked the style. A few weeks later, she phoned me up and asked 'What is wrong with these men?' Initially I didn't know what she was talking about. She then explained that she had given the manuscript to a young man to copy edit and he had started rewriting it. He, too, felt that the style should be changed. She told him to rub out all his pencil rewrites and edited the manuscript herself, doing what she, and we (co-authored by the late, Jill Louw), thought it needed – just a tidying up job. Women reading the book, *Disorderly Breasts* (Camden Press 1987), seem to have no problem with the style.

I was comfortable with the style of *Will, My Son* even if others found it threatening. It was a statement of what I thought and felt as well as a description of my experiences.

When I received my six free author's copies, my parents were among the first to receive a copy. They had been a source of great support throughout. They were, by coincidence, the first of the family to learn that Will was Down's Syndrome. The consultant had interrupted their first visit to me in hospital to tell me that my ten-day-old son was Down's Syndrome. My parents had been away at the birth. They had timed their holiday to be back in England for the expected date of delivery. Their, and our plans, had not anticipated that the delivery would happen six weeks prematurely. Ed had phoned them to tell them of the arrival of a new grandson and had reassured them, as we all thought, that mother and baby were fine. After receiving the shattering news about Will, the consultant told my parents at my request.

The next thing I remember was my parents coming in and immediately taking me in their arms and holding me. They too were visibly stunned and upset. My father went to phone Ed. He returned to the ward saying that Ed was out of the office but that he had left a message for him to phone the hospital immediately. We sat in the ward and I remember little of what was said.

From that moment on, my parents helped and supported us in a whole range of ways, both practically and emotionally. On the morning he died, they had decided to drive up to London as a result of a premonition that we might need them. They arrived at the hospital shortly after his death. Despite their own grief at the loss of a grandson, they simply moved into action, supporting us in our state of total shock. Therefore, giving them a copy of my book was very important to me.

Like any child taking home something they have done to their parents, there is apprehension, even when that child is 37 years old! Reading it I knew would be painful for them. As parents they had had to endure the pain of seeing their own child suffer so much hurt and being unable, as all parents wish, to magically take the pain away. They, too, had their own grief, having experienced the loss of two grandchildren. Their immediate response, though, was one of gentle praise. It was only with the passage of time that I realized just how much the book and its publication was to change my relationship with my mother.

Throughout my life, I have never doubted that both my parents loved me. I have, though, at times felt that they didn't understand me. A rift in understanding, I felt, came between my mother and myself in late adolescence and deepened throughout my years at university and all during my twenties. My mother committed her adult life to being a wife and mother. This is to give the impression that she was or is a conventional woman, but she wore trousers in the 1950s - baggy corduroy ones, which caused me acute embarrassment as a child - and is never happier than when tending a bonfire or doing her carpentry in the garage. Even so, I felt she had great difficulty in understanding my needs and aspirations. In particular, she showed little understanding of my interest in and commitment to work and my seeming lack of interest in pursuing marriage and motherhood. Underlying her attitude to me was disapproval of my lifestyle and of my choice to openly live with a man. We were never visibly hostile, but, equally, I knew that there were areas of evasion in our relationship that meant each keeping a certain emotional distance.

My relationship with my father was by nature different. He had actively supported and encouraged me to go to university, to stay on at university to do an MA and then enter the world of work. My father and I have always shared an interest in politics. Our political differences, when we have had them, have only been a question of degree. Feminism, mine and that of others, is inscrutable to him as it probably is to most other 85-year-old men, though, as a headmaster of a co-educational grammar school, he took the education of girls seriously. My lifestyle and my failure to get married and settle down appeared to concern him less than it did my mother. The concern he expressed was only in relation to my happiness and security.

Of course, from the moment Will was born, like most children who become parents, I found that the bond with my parents increased. From the outset, my father and mother supported Will and us, both emotionally and in terms of giving time and help. Around their grandchild there was a focus for greater mutual understanding.

My relationship with my mother became hugely easier. She was at ease with me in the role of mother. We could discuss his feeding, sleeping and playing patterns. I could discuss with her his handicap. After his death, I could be held by her. This focus of motherhood continued into my next pregnancy, through the birth and the first year of my daughter, Jessie's, life. Tension returned, however, when I felt a need to return to work. I knew my mother disapproved of a mother working who did not have an immediate obvious financial need to do so. For her, one's family should come first, without question.

Like many other women, my needs were to express myself both through work and through my personal relationships. No doubt, had my mother been of a different generation, she would also have felt these needs. At the outbreak of war, she was called up and drove an ambulance, which she thoroughly enjoyed, but, as an occupation, carpentry has always been her first love. In her garage turned workshop are bits of wood, lovingly kept for decades. Some wood, rescued from a German battleship being broken up in Edinburgh in 1948, has travelled with her through several moves around the country – 'You never know when you might need a piece just like that', she will say. Now, in her mid-seventies, periodically, she still goes off to woodworking classes. One of her most treasured possessions for years, until replaced by a more up-to-date model, was a Black and Decker drill, given to her in 1967 as a leaving present from the Girl Guides, which she had served as a District Commissioner.

Sadly, skill in carpentry is something I didn't learn from her. The Black and Decker drill was passed on to us and we still have it, though I have never used it. In these matters, Ed and I have a more conventional division of labour: I sew on the buttons and

Ed, when necessary, uses the drill. In the matter of working mothers, I was seen as the unconventional one. The first perceptible change in her attitude to me came after she had read *Will, My Son*. Nothing was said overtly, but the fact that she gave or lent copies to several people signalled to me that it was something she felt proud of. Over the years, she has continued to lend copies to people and relay to me their responses. Quietly, she has been a devoted supporter.

The change in our relationship is deeper, though, than just the fact that I wrote a book of which she could feel proud. The book, in a sense, was the coming together of my personal and political life. It was a merging of me as mother and me as a writer; the worlds of home and work meet in its pages. For the first time, I felt that my mother understood my need for these two worlds. She realized, too, that I had something to offer to the world outside of my immediate family. The tension around me working began to fade away and, with its fading, came a much closer relationship, one in which I could share with her my aspirations (and frustrations) about the world of work as well as the pleasures and pains of my domestic life. We even read many of the same books now and discuss them. Throughout my childhood I never remember seeing my mother reading anything other than *Woman's Own* and *Woman's Weekly* - her escape, as she would describe them. Now, though, we share our copies of Toni Morrison, Alice Walker, Jung Chang or sit down to watch together Jane Campion's film *Angel At My Table* and feel as women a shared response. Maybe this change in my relationship with my mother would have come about anyway, with the fullness of time, but, without *Will, My Son*, I am not *sure* that it would.

How the book changed the lives of others, mostly I will never know. Over the years, some have told me that it has made them think and question their attitudes. In one or two cases they have told me that it has actually changed their attitude.

One of my motives in seeking publication of the book was, indeed, to make people think, and I hoped it would also be part of a body of people who were writing, campaigning and putting change into practice. In looking to change wider social attitudes and practices, I did not think my book might influence someone at the very personal level of their own life. Therefore, I found it quite overwhelming when, in 1988, I received a letter from my Aunt, Aileen Constant. In it she told me that a friend of hers 'had become friendly with a young woman who was a talented art student, but decided she was being drawn to work with the handicapped – went to work in a home for children affected by Down's Syndrome and while there read your book on Will and was so impressed that she decided she would devote her life to them. She now has two adopted sons of six and a few months and is thinking about fostering a third.' My aunt's friend wondered if I wanted to meet this 'young woman'. Part of me wanted to respond and part of me didn't want to acknowledge responsibility for any influence my words may have had. It also made me feel uneasy in that this 'young woman' was clearly putting into practice what I advocated. Action speaks larger than words and writing, I felt and feel, is an easy cop out. At the time, I merely acknowledged the letter, but evaded the invitation.

In planning *this* book, I knew that going to see this 'young woman' was one of the loose ends of the legacy of *Will, My Son* that I had to explore. One afternoon in May 1993, I found myself, having written explaining my wish to meet her, knocking on the door of Lucy Baxter's home. My preconceptions of the kind of woman who adopts children with learning difficulties was quickly blown away when the door was opened by a tall, attractive young woman. It was yet another lesson to me of how many stereotypes of people we carry, unquestioningly, in our heads. After a slightly uneasy few minutes, we settled down to talk for a good four hours, interrupted by picking up her younger son, Otto, from school and the return of James from his school.

I asked Lucy a gamut of questions, some very personal, and she replied to them all with a generous openness. Many of my questions were about her experience of attitudes to children with learning difficulties and the facilities that are provided for them. I was exploring, for a chapter of this book, the changes that have taken place over the years. The other area of questions was more personal to her and to me. I was particularly interested in the experiences that had led her to adopt Down's Syndrome children.

In the course of the afternoon, it emerged that Lucy had, after studying briefly at an art school, moved into working with children with learning difficulties. While working, she increasingly felt that being a 'service worker' was not the way she could best give of her abilities and her care. On a trip to the West Country, she met someone who had adopted Down's Syndrome children and from them she learned that adoption could be possible for her as a single parent. Her commitment to Down's Syndrome children had come from working with them. Lucy then set about to change her life. She became committed to providing care for the Down's Syndrome children she would adopt.

James, now 11, was her first adoption. He came to her aged four, finding with Lucy a safe haven after three years of disrupted care and abuse. It emerged after the adoption had been processed that James was also autistic. The latter you would not have known witnessing his return from school that day. A taxi delivered him home. He came into the room with his mother, sat on her knee and gave her a big cuddle and, smiling, gave her several kisses. Witnessing this, beside me, was five-year-old Otto, who expressed a little normal sibling jealousy by throwing a toy across the room to attract his mother's attention. My first sight of Otto had been in the school playground. Otto attends the local 'mainstream' infant school and I went with Lucy to pick him up from there. This tiny, smiling, affectionate little boy appeared with a friend. I couldn't help thinking of another tiny, smiling boy that I had hoped one day I would stand and wait for in a normal school playground.

Lucy's house and garden immediately give you the feeling of a place lived in and used by children. In the garden is a wonderful, large, yellow wendy house, a trampoline and other play equipment. Inside there is all the normal paraphernalia of a house inhabited by two boys. After both boys had returned home, Lucy and I continued talking and talking. The boys sat glued to a video, each coming into the sitting room from time to time for a little attention. In this atmosphere of 'family normality' it was hard to remember that the origins of this family unit were in no way 'normal'. In fact, its creation turns normal social attitudes on their head. Most see having a Down's Syndrome child as something they would not willingly choose. Lucy, who could have chosen otherwise, saw adopting a child with Down's Syndrome as something she positively wanted. Lucy set out to create a family, to choose Down's Syndrome children and to offer them her love and care. The path of parenthood is not always easy and with James she has had, and still has, many problems, but sitting there in her house you cannot but feel that James and Otto have been given a chance to experience love and affection and are supported by a mother who is dedicated to helping them develop to their full potential.

I asked about her decision to adopt rather than foster. Lucy was very clear about this. She wanted to bring her children up in her own way and not have to bring them up according to the dictates of a committee of service workers. Indeed, being able to do it her way was part of Lucy's reason for choosing to move out of employment as a service worker and into parenthood.

Shortly before I left, Lucy produced an obviously well-read copy of *Will, My Son* and asked me to sign it. Signing it seemed such an inadequate expression of my feelings of gratitude to her. It was then she told me that she had read many other books by parents, but *Will, My Son* had been special. 'He left such a deep impression on me', she said and added, 'There was no other book like it for me'. Will's legacy has, indeed, been great.

TOO DEEP FOR TEARS

One of my reasons for not responding to my Aunt's initial invitation to meet Lucy Baxter was that, after writing *Will, My Son*, I withdrew from any direct involvement in issues to do with Down's Syndrome. My withdrawal was motivated by two feelings. One, quite instinctive, was to do with my emotional survival. To be around the issues or around people with Down's Syndrome was to keep me in the past. I felt, in particular, that to be close to children with Down's Syndrome would have drawn me into trying to recreate the life of Will through the lives of others. I felt I needed to live in the present and to concern myself with the present and the future. Therefore, I did not seek out contact with people with Down's Syndrome or information about them. Whenever I saw a Down's Syndrome child or person I, of course, would watch them. My daughter accuses me, often rightfully, of staring at people in general. I know I have consciously stared whenever I have seen someone with Down's Syndrome. My stare is one that is loaded with the pain of grief and of what might have been. Caught by the recipient of my stare, I look away and think, 'if only they knew why I am staring'. Besides needing to live in the present, I also eschewed involvement with any campaigns for and on behalf of people with Down's Syndrome because I was always aware that I never had to live with the ongoing problems and struggles of parenting a child with Down's Syndrome. I was conscious that people might say, 'It is all very well for her to talk, but she doesn't have to deal with it'.

Although I consciously avoided involvement, there has always been a part of me that has wondered what has been happening in the world into which I was so briefly and passionately plunged. On the back cover of *Will, My Son*, the publisher wrote, 'Sarah Boston uses personal experience to raise important issues about our response to the handicapped and our treatment of both them and their families. She calls for radical change, particularly from doctors and social workers, and affirms the right of all handicapped people to an equal chance of life'. Returning to these areas after years of absence, I found that, although I brought a historical perspective, none of my original concern and passion had been diluted by the years.

Writing this book was a way of finding an excuse that would legitimate to myself and to others this journey of discovery. I am also aware that, just as I wrote *Will, My Son* when I had reached a level of emotional safety, I return again to the subject at a particular stage of my life. On 14 February 1993, Will would have been 18, his childhood years completed. My daughter, now 16, is on the brink of adulthood, so my years of mothering as the prime focus of my life are coming to an end. I enter a new phase and, as I do, I look back. Looking back is a way of marking a stage to enable one to move forward.

Grief is not something I have been absent from and can choose to return to. Although this book is not motivated by a desperate need to try and transfer experiences from my head to paper it is, as *Will, My Son* was, informed by grief. Four, nearly five years, after Will's death, to write of my grief was, I felt, socially acceptable. Eighteen years after his death, though, I am deeply conscious that most people in society think that such things should have been left well behind. Yet, such experiences are never left behind in the heart and memory of the survivor; they inform your life.

I wrote this introduction confidently assuming my mother would be alive to read it. I had wanted to express, to her, my gratitude for the love and support she always gave me. Sadly she will never read this, nor any of my words, again. On the 28 January 1994 my mother, Jo Boston, died.

1 / The medical profession

From the moment Will was born until his death, the medical profession played a central role in his, and our, lives. Much of *Will, My Son* described and commented on our interaction with 'the professionals'. My purpose in doing so was to raise questions about the attitudes and practices of the medical profession with the hope of being part of a body of people arguing for change. Eighteen years on, I wondered whether any of these arguments had filtered through to professional practice.

Before starting on this book, my nephew, then a medical student at St George's, phoned me with the information that, on one of his courses, he had been given a book list which included *Will, My Son*. The course required students to pick a book (that was not a medical textbook) or a film about people with learning difficulties and discuss it with the class. My response to this information was to say that I would love to be a 'fly on the wall' and listen to the discussion relating to *Will, My Son*.

At the time, I knew such a request would be seen as an indulgence on my behalf. Writing this book, though, gave me a respectable reason for approaching St George's and asking if I could attend such a seminar. I thought that finding out the attitudes of medical students - the doctors of the future - would be a good place to start my research. The response from St George's, in the person of Dr Jane Bernal, was very generous. Dr Bernal explained that the format of the session had changed, but that she would be quite happy to devote one session in the second-year clinical students' course on the psychiatry of disability to my book and to a discussion of the issues it raises. I was invited to participate in any way I wished. My wish, I told her, was to listen. My interest was how much attitudes had changed and whether or not our concerns about the issues raised in the book were of concern to the doctors of tomorrow.

As I drove across London to St George's for the session, I felt apprehensive. On arrival, Dr Jane Bernal apologized for not being totally organized, but she had come into work that morning to find that her secretary was in a state of understandably extreme anxiety and anger. The previous evening, the secretary had been visiting her mother who was in one of the wards. During her visit, a consultant had told her quite bluntly that he might have to amputate her mother's foot. This information had been conveyed directly to her across the bed in which her mother was lying. This situation put into immediate sharp focus the issues – issues of sensitivity and respect – that we would be discussing with the students.

As we entered the classroom and I unpacked my tape recorder, I felt distinctly nervous. I watched the students as they meandered in. To me they looked very young, were conventionally dressed and, to my surprise, the group was about equally divided in terms of gender. A few ethnic minorities were also represented. At the beginning, my presence clearly unnerved Dr Jane Bernal, but, as she settled in to leading the discussion, the effect of my presence appeared to diminish. Not knowing the class, I could not gauge how much my presence affected the students and their discussion.

After the normal explanations, introductions and a request made on my behalf to tape record the session, Dr Jane Bernal started by reading the title of my book and the subtitle, *The Life and Death of a Mongol Child,* commenting that she assumed that 'the word "mongol" was probably chosen very carefully in order to shock, in order to make you think what sort of person it is that other people call mongols'. She told the students that 'The word Down's Syndrome was around in the seventies as it is now, but the word mongol was and is the word the general public know and use'. I sat there wishing that the subtitle had been chosen for such commendable reasons. The use of the word 'mongol' on the front cover was the only thing that the publisher and I had disagreed about. During Will's life, I had been on a journey of discovery. The book charts this discovery. In the early part, I use the word I knew – and that used to me by the paediatrician who first broke the news to me - mongol. By the time Will was two months' old, I had learned that Down's Syndrome was the appropriate term and changed my usage, both in describing Will to others at the time and reflected this change in the book. From Chapter 5 onwards, I write of Down's Syndrome. The publishers, however, felt that the term mongol was the popularly understood word and so it should be used on the front cover. I did not fight their argument, merely signalling that I felt uncomfortable about it. With hindsight, for a publishing company that prided itself on being 'politically correct' (before this phrase had been coined), their decision to use the term mongol was to stoop to the worst kind of popularism. I regret I let it happen.

After commenting on the word mongol, Dr Bernal launched into the first issue - breaking the news that a child is Down's Syndrome. It was very strange to sit there listening to my words being read, extremely well, by someone else to a classroom full of students. Dr Bernal explained that it was ten days after Will's birth that the news was broken to me.

The sister, the consultant paediatrician, and his junior registrar came over to my bed. The sister pulled the curtains round my bed. I knew then that whatever they were going to say to me was going to be serious. I sat on the edge of my bed, the consultant on a chair immediately opposite me, the registrar sat to my right and the sister stood further to my right and outside of my easy vision. The consultant started talking. I remember little of his precise words except that somewhere in those words was the fact that my child was a mongol. 'You had been uneasy, you had suspected that something was wrong, hadn't you?' he said, almost appealing to me, as if the fact that I had already suspected that something was wrong would soften the blow. I admitted that I had, but I had never suspected that something was so fundamentally and completely wrong with Will. I started to cry before he had even told me exactly what it was and I continued crying . . .

The consultant was obviously finding the task of telling me about Will a difficult one, although he must have had considerable experience. The junior registrar was even more uncomfortable. I could see him sitting there hardly daring to look at me and evading my eyes whenever I looked at him. In fact he was a kind, gentle man but both he and his consultant were obviously unschooled in handling such situations.

By the students' response, it would seem paediatricians are still largely unschooled in handling such matters. Having read this extract, Dr Bernal asked, 'How exceptional is that experience now?' The response from one student was, 'I think it is probably quite common that situation because, as I understand it, a paediatrician won't have that much psychiatric training. I mean he might only have done what we do - 11 weeks and that is it'.

A discussion then followed as to how the 'breaking of the news' could have been handled more sensitively. The students felt that my partner, Ed, should have been there so that we were told together. Another suggested that the child should have been present. In my case, this would have been problematic as Will, having been born prematurely was still in the neonatal intensive care unit. However, I could imagine how much the presence of Will could have changed the scene. If the paediatrician, or even the sister or junior registrar, had given Will attention by smiling and talking to him in the way most people do with babies, the messages conveyed, not just in words but in body language, would have been so much more positive. In their actions they would have been expressing their acceptance of him as a person.

Such news should be broken, the students thought, in a private place, with a door that could be shut. Curtains are, as any patient in a ward knows, not soundproof. The students also discussed the question of the allocation of time. They felt that, in general, a lot of time should be allocated by the consultant and other medical personnel to the breaking of such news and that time should be made for further discussions.

With a little prodding from Dr Bernal, the students between them in fact came up with the main guidelines given by Dr Sheila Jupp in a pamphlet entitled *Making the Right Start: A practical manual to help break the news to families when their baby has been born with a disability*, published in 1992. The July/August 1993 issue of *Mencap News* reports that a working party had just drawn up guidelines for the breaking of 'bad news' to parents. The key guidance points that the Mencap working party hope the medical profession will take on board when having to break news to parents about a baby's disability are privacy, time, not being alone, the allocation of time for further discussions and the provision of information. The tone of the article, however, is one informed as much by a fear of not upsetting the medical profession as by the demand that the needs of parents are considered. 'The Guidelines', they state, 'were never intended to tell anybody how to do their job, but to act as a way of ensuring that the method in which a parent or parents are helped at such a crucial time is consistent.' Several 'understanding' references are made to the problems busy consultants face in finding adequate time and a private place in which to break news. Given that the consequences of this first consultation can be so great - for life, literally - surely one should simply *demand* good practice.

Dr Sheila Jupp obviously feels, as a Consultant Clinical Psychologist, more confident in telling the medical profession how to do their job. She writes, 'First, professionals need to understand that breaking the news in a balanced and effective way is not easy to accomplish. An impression of what is said and done at this time, if not a full transcript of what happened, will almost certainly be imprinted on the memories of parents for the rest of their lives. Therefore, the disclosure itself, requires a good deal of thought, skill and planning, if it is to give parents the true consideration that they expect and deserve'.

These two sets of very recent guidelines reveal that, clearly, there is still a long way to go in educating the medical profession in more sensitive ways of communicating such news to parents. Indeed, the fact that in the nineties people are still trying to 'educate' doctors in more sensitive ways of communicating information reveals just how slow progress in some areas can be.

Charles Hannam, a father of a Down's Syndrome child and author of *Parents and Mentally Handicapped Children*, (Penguin 1975) wrote in 1975, 'A survey conducted in London in 1964, quoted in the introduction to Barbara Furneaux's *The Special Child*, (Penguin 1973) stated that "in many instances the communication of the discovery of mental defect was handled badly". Sadly I found this still to be true'. I also, in 1993, sadly found it still to be true.

The Down's Syndrome Association, though aware that they hear mainly the horror stories, still hear horror stories. They hear stories of parents being told of their child's disability in thoughtless and insensitive ways. In 1975, Charles Hannam commented, after recounting the horror stories he had heard, 'One wonders whether the telling of the news should be left to doctors at all'. If acquiring the skill of a doctor leaves neither the time nor the inclination to develop skills in communication, then perhaps the job *should* be given to those who do have the time and the inclination to develop these skills. One doctor said to me, when I was raising questions about the lack of communication skills in the medical profession, 'Would you rather be operated on by a surgeon who was a skilled surgeon or one who was a skilled communicator'. Put like this, of course one would choose the skill in surgery. However, the problem is not one of either or, it is a problem of attitude. Many patients feel doctors do not even see that there is a need to try to communicate in clear and sensitive ways.

The importance of how the news is broken cannot be underestimated as the emotional consequences are often long term and the memory, as Sheila Jupp and others have found, is for life. I wrote the following in *Will, My Son*.

> Besides 'thinking big' in those first few hours, I also went through time and time again the events of the afternoon. That same mother who had told us about her reaction to the fact her child was a mongol also remarked on how vividly, even 13 years later, she remembered how she was told.

I still have total recall of the scene in the hospital ward. Mostly it remains tucked away in my mind. Twice in the past six months the memory has been set into replay. The first happened while watching a themed evening of programmes about childbirth on BBC 2. Running throughout the evening between programmes were short 'to camera' accounts by parents of childbirth. Suddenly, I found I was sitting riveted to my chair. A silence fell on Ed, Jessie and myself as we realized what was being described by the woman on the screen was how she had been told her child was Down's Syndrome and of her immediate reaction. She recounted, 'I just couldn't think what Down's Syndrome was. My mind just went blank. I just couldn't believe I was hearing what he said. He was so negative about it. I thought that I had got a vegetable that wouldn't walk or talk'. Once home with her baby, things started going very wrong. 'I really felt like killing my daughter. That seemed like the solution. I'd get rid of her. I'd get rid of the problem.' She then went on to tell of how she came to accept her daughter, helped by the loving support of her mother and of her father who had said, 'Well, she is just a little baby'. The final image of this short piece was the woman, smiling, with her two daughters. Ed's comment was 'It seems like doctors haven't changed much – I mean, her daughter is only a few years old. It can't have happened that long ago'. As I listened to this mother's story, vivid memories of the day I was told came back and I began to cry. Jessie sat with us, uncomfortably aware that what she had just heard touched deep emotions in her own parents.

The second time the memory came to the forefront of my mind was when I attending the same hospital that Will had been born in for minor surgery. I had to pass the old part of the hospital where the maternity ward is. I looked up. There was the corner window that my bed had stood by and in front of that very window the paediatrician had sat to break the news to me. I needed no continuity person with a polaroid camera and a notebook to make sure every detail of the scene could be remembered accurately for the next day's filming. In my mind I looked in and replayed, in precise detail, that afternoon, 18 years later.

My clarity of memory is not exceptional. In discussing the question of how parents are told, Dr Jane Bernal explained to the students, 'The reason why I am laying such stress on it is because what it says here [pointing to *Will, My Son*] really is true. People who have looked at the parents of children with disabilities who have now grown up and are in their twenties and thirties can remember every word that they heard the paediatrician say. That isn't necessarily what the paediatrician thinks they said, but, what the mothers remember, they remember with great clarity'.

Dr Bernal elaborated this point by referring to research work done by Janet Carr, one of her colleagues at St George's. Janet Carr asked mothers in the first year of the life of their child what they remembered about being told of their child's disability. She then went back and asked these same mothers what they remembered when their child was 21 and found that the accounts were almost identical. Janet Carr's research confirms that vivid recall of 'the scene' is common. 'It really is something that hangs around and colours both how people view their children and the medical profession thereafter', Dr Bernal emphasized to the students.

Only one student interjected at this point. The student commented, 'But isn't it also true that parents often remember very different things to what the paediatrician thinks or says he or she said. That first admission of something being wrong with the child is just remembered by the parents as they remember it regardless of what happened, so maybe there isn't much the paediatrician can do'. What the student failed to take on board was that parents pick up on two forms of language in such a situation. One is the actual words and, in a stunned state, others no doubt, like myself, may well 'hear' little except the hard core of the information. No parent I have met or read about failed to understand the central message – disability. The second form of communication is body language. The tone of the voice, the demeanour of the paediatrician, the setting, the pacing – all contribute positively or negatively to the message being communicated. Parents who have experienced being told such news *know* that there *is* 'much the paediatrician can do'.

Later in the seminar, the subject of parents' responses to the news of their child's disability was returned to. Dr Bernal explained that, 'We have talked a lot about what the medical profession have or haven't done. Because (a) the book really does talk a lot about that. Certainly, when I first read the book I was a paediatrician on a neonatal intensive care unit and I was very struck by how much it had to say about the sorts of ways that I and people like me behaved, but also because (b) you're doctors, you are going to be doctors and it is important that you think of these things'.

Dr Bernal then reminded the students of earlier seminars, when they had been introduced to the emotional responses of people after receiving bad news of different kinds. She told the students that in my book there was a lot of anger and commented, 'it is mostly anger, I think, which is quite appropriately directed at the medical profession for saying things that weren't helpful. But', she added 'anger is also part of the grieving process and I think there is a practice point for all of us'. The practice point being, she went on to explain, that there is now a received wisdom taught to medical students and professional carers that people following bereavement or the shock of being told such things as their baby having a disability go through different stages of emotional response. Indeed, Sheila Jupp includes in her booklet *Making The Right Start* two models, very similar, of the stages of a parent's response. The first, a graph (Copyright American Academy of Pediatrics 1975), shows a 'Hypothetical model of the sequence of normal parental reactions to the birth of a child with congenital malformations', and details the intensity and time duration of these reactions. In Britain, Cliff Cunningham has also studied parents' responses. He developed what he calls his model of 'Psychic Crisis at Disclosure of Handicap'. In this, Cliff Cunningham details the phases (shock, reaction, adaptation, orientation and 'crisis over') and, in relation to these phases, he lists how they might manifest themselves in the parents' behaviour. The model goes further and also lists the support parents may need from different professionals at each stage. Sheila Jupp wisely comments that Cunningham's model is 'intended to guide professional considerations of counselling and is not to be imposed upon parents, since some people will not necessarily display all these stages or reactions and many will oscillate between phases at different times and in different contexts'.

The results of this work can be very useful in helping parents through the first period of time. It is particularly helpful when, as Cliff Cunningham has done, it is used to guide the medical profession and other carers in the kinds of help, information, support and understanding that parents might need. Unfortunately, in the teaching of the stages of emotional responses, particularly in relation to bereavement (which I shall discuss later in this book), cruder versions have often become gospel. People are expected to go through each 'stage' in an orderly fashion and are deemed not to have 'dealt' with their trauma unless they have completed this course of self-therapy satisfactorily.

In counselling the students on this question, Dr Jane Bernal also wisely cautioned them against taking a crude, self-defensive position in relation to the parents' responses, particularly their anger. 'There were a lot of people', she said, 'when I was in paediatrics who had read this stuff about bereavement and about when somebody is told their child has a disability. They have learned - "they *are* going to feel guilty, they *are* going to feel angry". It is very easy to blame things', Dr Bernal cautioned, 'on somebody else's psycho-pathology that are actually *your* misdeeds. It is easy to say 'Well, *I* didn't tell that mother wrongly. The problem is *she's* angry with the medical profession. We all know that is part of the grieving process". She went on to say, 'You don't want to take more responsibility than you have to; you don't want to be totally distressed and unable to function because a parent is so angry and wishes to sue you; but, equally, you do need to consider each time when a parent is angry with you whether or not you have or haven't done anything to deserve that anger rather than assuming, as some people do, having heard that stuff about bereavement, that it is necessarily the parent who is at fault rather than yourselves'.

This point led Dr Bernal to explore with the students the process of professionalizing medical students, moving them from being feeling human creatures to desensitized doctors. She commented on how much sensitivity medical students displayed in a workshop she regularly held with students and a parent of a disabled child. 'Yet', she went on, 'somehow it continues to be difficult for doctors who are qualified to do things as sensitively as the medical students do in that seminar'. Dr Bernal then described to the students her most recent experience of a doctor's insensitivity - her secretary being told her mother's foot might have to be amputated. Not surprisingly, this subject - the process of desensitizing medical students - triggered the most lively and impassioned comments from the group. The students felt that they had had to develop a hard shell to protect themselves, not just from the distressing situations they had to deal with, but in order to enable them to cope with the treatment they received from their superiors in the course of training. The students, with one voice, described this educational approach as 'learning by humiliation'. One student complained that, 'As a medical student, we get insulted quite a lot by all the members of staff, by doctors and everybody and that is how you learn'. The student then added, 'It is mostly the consultants who insult us'. There were general murmurs of agreement, particularly with the last comment. These consultants are for better – or, perhaps, in terms of teaching – for worse the people the students acknowledged as their 'role models'. Paediatricians and psychiatrists were agreed to be, on the whole, a more considerate species, whereas surgeons were often deemed to be behavioural monsters. Dr Bernal asked if surgeons were born with, 'a personality disorder', or, 'does something happen to them, and when does it happen?'

The stress of the work was seen as one reason, and the inevitable process of 'emotional hardening' that it was felt doctors needed to undergo in order to deal with stress and human suffering. A young man talked of his distress at witnessing his first death and of his concern, too, that, by the time he had witnessed a few deaths, he no longer felt the same distress. 'You would break down if you sympathized with every patient', one student commented, but another quickly chipped in, 'You don't need sympathy, basic courtesy will do'.

One student pointed out that patients tended to remember the bad experiences they had had with doctors rather than the good ones. Research does show that patients often quickly gloss over the times their interactions with the medical profession have been good, with passing comments like 'Oh she/he was very good', but they detail, at length, the bad experiences.

The comment relating to patients' memories triggered Dr Bernal to return the discussion to *Will, My Son* and to the fact that she thought I had been very fair in offering praise as well as criticism. 'The star of it', Dr Bernal stated, 'After Will [I felt a sensation of pride run through me to hear my son referred to as a 'star'] was Doctor Z.' The reason she gave for Dr Z's special place in my life was that Dr Z had not just shown deep sensitivity to my feelings, but had also shared something of herself as a human being with me. Dr Z was the doctor from the hospital's Home Care Unit who was assigned to care for Will when he was allowed home, aged six weeks. I first met Dr Z the day before taking Will home.

> She questioned me about his birth, feeding and other problems. She then asked me what my plans were for when I took him home. I explained that for the first week Ed would be at home too, so that I should be able to cope with the practical problems. I also explained that I was very nervous. After six weeks of always having professionals on hand for help and advice the prospect of being on my own frightened me. Dr Z then asked me when I would like visiting at home. The question rather surprised me. Most doctors tell you when and whether they will visit you. She then rather tentatively said 'I don't want to intrude on you and your husband during your first week at home with William'.
>
> . . .
>
> For the first time in my experience a doctor had actually shown real sensitivity about a human, family situation. It impressed me deeply. Later many more things about Dr Z were to impress me.

One student noted that Dr Z in gently, where appropriate, bringing some of herself as a human being to the relationship of professional and client was 'breaking down the traditional doctor patient stand'. The students registered unease at this thought and at Dr Bernal's suggestion that, as a doctor, it is, 'OK to let your patients know you are a human being'. One student felt that Dr Z could be seen by me as 'nicer' because she hadn't been involved in the initial telling of bad news. I made one of my only interjections at this point, saying that Dr Z was, indeed, involved later in breaking bad news to me. It was Dr Z who first heard Will's heart murmur and had had to break this news to me. It was true that Dr Z was better placed, as a home care unit doctor, visiting me and Will in my home to give me time and consideration. She was not having to work within the strictures of hospital routines and hospital buildings, but Dr Z's qualities were not just products of time and place, they were products of a particular attitude to her role as a doctor and as a human being.

Dr Bernal saw, as I do, Dr Z as 'a positive role model'. I was not convinced that many of the students were as sure.

There was unanimity in their view that doctors should treat people, other professionals and patients, with 'basic courtesy', but they were clearly uneasy about going any further.

Safety for these students lies in the traditional doctor–patient relationship. For many reasons, they see it as dangerous and emotionally threatening to step outside it. They know they have emotions and look to the one model they have to protect themselves. The training of medical students is based on the premiss, 'professional doctors don't have emotions'. Their predecessors have built up a professional code that works as an emotional defence system for the profession. What may be upsetting situations are handled by the profession in ways that best protect them and their feelings. They are not ways that best help the patient or the relatives of the patient. Ultimately, however, all the parties suffer. The clients are not just emotionally hurt, but are left alienated from the medical profession. The doctor–patient relationship suffers and the doctor and patient individually suffer.

Another training approach would be to work from the premiss that recognizes doctors as human beings who may have strong, complicated and sometimes painful emotions (including anger). Just as the emotional responses of parents who have just been told of their child's disability have been studied, research should be done into the emotional stages medical students go through from day one to being fully qualified practitioners. Lists could then be drawn up of their needs, and support given to help steer them through to qualifying as doctors *and* human beings. One can only feel that such an approach would be of benefit to them and their emotional well-being as well as be of benefit to the patient. In the absence of such an approach, one can only hope that students now go out with a little more training and a little more sensitivity. A little imagination would not go amiss either. One wonders if doctors ever imagine themselves in a situation and stop to think how they would feel or react.

BAD NEWS?

Having discussed how best disclosure can be made to parents that their child has a disability, Dr Bernal dropped in the big question. She led in to it gently, by reminding the students that, in their first clinical year, her department had done a session with them on 'breaking bad news'. 'I wonder', she asked, 'if this really *is* bad news?' In this simple question she was probing the heart of their attitudes. One student remembered watching a video in the session in which the breaking of the news to a parent that their child was Down's Syndrome was included. Another remembered a mother of a Down's Syndrome child who had talked to the students in a seminar on learning disabilities. The parent had stressed to the students that it *wasn't* bad news, that it shouldn't be put across as bad news, but just as news about the child - that the child is slightly different. Dr Bernal suggested that maybe it was neutral news, news about difference. Despite having just been reminded of what a parent had told them, indeed *stressed* to them, in a previous seminar on learning disabilities, one student quickly cut in and said, 'I can't really agree with that'. To sounds of agreement from others he went on, 'You can present it as neutral news, but, really, I think anyone who says it is neutral news is ridiculous. What parent would want their child to have a learning disability? No one would. It doesn't mean they can't love their child, but, in reality, it *is* bad news. I think to be going "Oh my goodness, I am so sorry" isn't very helpful, but, on the other hand, to be chirpy about it wouldn't be very helpful'. This statement reflected the general attitude of the class.

It probably also reflects the attitude of most people. All expectant parents - I have never met an exception - hope that their baby will be normal and healthy. Finding that it is any way otherwise always requires an adjustment. Expectations go deeper still, though. When I was pregnant with Will, I did not realize that I was carrying not just an unborn child, but also an unconscious fantasy about that child. In one word 'mongol', I realized I had had a fantasy and that, in saying this word, the fantasy was shattered.

Whilst Will was still in the incubator, before we knew of his mongolism, I remember Ed looking at one of his tiny feet and joking about how that foot might be the foot which scored the winning goal for Arsenal in a cup final twenty odd years hence. It was the kind of comment half joking, half fanciful, part wishing, parents make particularly of tiny babies. In the first few weeks after we knew about Will's handicap it was the kind of comment we did not make. We were painfully aware of all the things he definitely would not do. It left little room for us to fantasise about greatness and glory.

Of course, being an inveterate dreamer, I quickly developed *new* fantasies for my new baby. Fantasies have a habit of accommodating themselves to reality.

The question is whether or not, in the light of human expectation, let alone the prevailing social attitudes, the news that a baby has a disability is, or ever can, be neutral. The giver of the information and the receiver of this information come to the situation already informed by their own attitudes. Both parties bring to the situation a notion of whether or not such information is 'bad news' or a 'disclosure about difference'. What is brought, in terms of attitudes, to the situation will have a profound influence on the response to it.

What attitudes my consultant paediatrician brought to this moment of disclosure were very much a reflection of the dominant attitudes of the time – 1975. He was breaking to me 'bad news', of that I am sure he had no doubt. I assume also that, as a paediatrician, he had a list in his head of the possible physical complications that can accompany Down's Syndrome – heart disease being the most serious. His view of Down's Syndrome was, I am sure, informed by a medical textbook. Besides the textbook image, doctors see patients because they are ill. Their view of a condition is coloured by illness, unless they have had non-professional contact. In the case of Down's Syndrome, this view had been further coloured by the fact that the average life expectancy, historically, had been brief. Early statistics revealed a pre-World-War-II life expectancy of nine years. By the late fifties/early sixties, statistics showed that life expectancy had doubled to about 18 years. Given the age of my consultant paediatrician, he had probably studied during this period and was informed by a view that Down's Syndrome children, on average, did not live for long. Going on past evidence, not future prognosis, he probably thought my child would have a short life. This expectation, not expressed, no doubt informed his response to one of my first questions.

> I didn't at that stage ask many questions. I was too dazed even to think of any, but I did ask 'What will happen to him when he grows up?' Sitting there on the bed a few minutes after having been told that Will was a mongol I somehow thought that I could cope with the prospect of his childhood but what then? The consultant muttered something about sheltered workshops and things being better than they were.

Maybe he was aware of the fact that, by then, the seventies, the most recent statistics revealed an increased life expectancy to an average of 30 years. What he could not have known was that, by 1985, life expectancy of Down's Syndrome people would have increased to 40 years *plus* - the plus leaving open the expectation that there will be a further upward revision of this figure. Indeed, life expectancy of Down's Syndrome has so increased that a new medical complication has been added to the list associated with Down's Syndrome-Alzheimer's disease.

In his response to my question about Will's 'adult life', at least my consultant left the door open for hope. Later, I was to appreciate this.

> The consultant did not tell me, as so many other parents of mongol children were told (and a few still are), that they should not expect their child ever to do anything. He left Will's potentialities quite open, basically by evading the issue.

It was shocking to find out that the above statement could also have been written in 1993. The Down's Syndrome Association find that, often, 'At best parents are given no information and at worst the information they are given is ill-informed and inaccurate'. Some parents are still told at the outset that they should not expect their child to achieve anything. Although the medical profession has gained more and more medical knowledge over the years, it has shown a deep reluctance to acquire knowledge about the *social* development of children with Down's Syndrome. The Association has an information pack that they send to maternity wards. Knowing whether or not this information pack ends up with the parents who have need of it, though, is hard to monitor. From the stories about the ignorance of paediatricians, it is clear they do not end up being read by the professionals. Now, as then, however, no information is better than misinformation.

Whether my paediatrician evaded the issue because he genuinely felt uncertain of Will's potentialities or whether he did not, at that point, want to burden me with more 'bad news', I can only guess. His behaviour would lead me towards the latter interpretation. In contrast to the registrar and the sister in the neonatal intensive care unit, the consultant never showed any warmth or direct communication with Will. I remember the sister chatting away to Will with humour and affection as she helped me bath and feed him. The registrar, too, responded to Will as a baby who needed emotional as well as physical care. 'He'll need feeding and loving and playing with just like a normal child', he told me when I asked him whether or not there was anything special I should do in terms of care when I took Will home. In the difference between the registrar and the consultant there were obviously differences in their own individual personalities, but there was also a difference in age. The registrar was a generation younger. My consultant had undoubtedly been taught by paediatricians who viewed the birth of a Down's Syndrome child as a tragedy, but one that would be, for the parents, short-lived. Their advice usually was, 'forget about this one, get on with conceiving the next', unless the mother was elderly or had already had several children, in which case, they would have advised her against having any more.

When I learned later of how other parents were told, I appreciated that my consultant approached meeting me that afternoon with more enlightened attitudes than his predecessors and many of his contemporaries. He also came to this meeting with the confirmation of Will's Down's Syndrome contained in the results of a test that showed that Will had 47 chromosomes instead of 46. It was only in the late fifties that, finally, the cause of Down's Syndrome - an extra chromosome had been identified. Another term for Down's Syndrome is Trisomy 21. In the nucleus of each normal human cell, there are 46 chromosomes, which are paired - the chromosomes being numbered 1 to 22 and the additional pair being the sex chromosome (xx for female and xy for male). In Trisomy 21 there is an extra number 21 chromosome attached to the twenty-first pair, making 3 instead of 2 in every cell. Standard Trisomy 21 accounts for about 90 to 95 per cent of Down's Syndrome cases. Mosaic Trisomy 21, found in a tiny percentage of cases, is when there is a mixture of trisomic cells and normal cells. Translocation Trisomy 21, again a small percentage of cases, is when the extra chromosome 21 has attached to another pair of chromosomes. However, how the extra chromosome sneaks in at the moment of conception when the sperm meets the egg is not known, and there appears to be some way to go, in terms of research, before the answer is found.

By 1975, thankfully, notions long held by many, including the medical profession, that Down's Syndrome was caused in some way by parental sin could no longer be sustained. Science had forced change. This change helped us.

> We never thought to try to conceal his mongolism. This was made easier for us as neither of us had any religious belief in the 'sins of the fathers', 'reincarnation', the 'will of God' or the will of any other supernatural power. We both knew that it was simply a genetic accident, the result of Will having an extra chromosome. But whilst I accepted it and did not feel guilty, I did feel a failure.

Although medically well-informed, the feedback I received both that afternoon and at further meetings was that my consultant paediatrician had little 'social' knowledge of Down's Syndrome. His image was probably socially as ignorant and as negative as mine. What I brought to the moment of disclosure was ignorance. Of this I wrote.

At the time I knew nothing about mongolism or mongol babies. I realised it meant mental handicap, mental retardation, subnormality. An image flashed before my mind of a child with an abnormally large head, the slanted eyes associated with mongolism and a vacant face. That was my image of mongolism culled, I'm not sure from where, but largely from ignorance.

It is hard to know where my image came from, except that it was probably typical of the general population in 1975. I had had no personal contact with anyone with Down's Syndrome, not even a nodding acquaintance. They were not, with very few exceptions, out in the streets, in shops, on public transport or in children's playgrounds. It was still the era when almost all Down's Syndrome people were segregated in special schools, special homes and in special holiday homes. Images were few and far between. The few that were available were negative. They were of sad, 'mentally defective' children who required our charity; their parents required our pity and their carers our admiration. It is hardly surprising that I brought to this meeting a negative image and responded with stunned awe at the situation I suddenly found we and our child were in.

I had hoped to find that, in the nineties, each side would bring more enlightened and better-informed attitudes to the moment of disclosure. It seems that, sadly, change is very slow in happening. Changing the images that we carry in our heads, which have been imprinted, both consciously and unconsciously, from what is around, has been a central concern for those campaigning for change. Between 1975 and 1993 there have been conscious moves to change the imagery, though how much of this has filtered through to the general public and the medical profession is hard to measure.

The literature, and there was very little about, that I managed to find about Down's Syndrome in 1975 had limited imagery. Only three publications included any images. One pamphlet by MIND, entitled *Your Mongol Baby*, had two photos of babies, which were both positive. Another, *Improving Babies with Down's Syndrome*, written by Rex Brinkworth and Dr Joseph Collins, had several photos, but, as the aim of the book was to introduce parents to various routines that would give mental and physical stimulation to the baby, most of the photos were illustrative. The only pamphlet that gave positive imagery and hope was one that had been published in America by the National Association for Retarded Citizens (1974) and was written by David Pitt. The images stretch from babyhood to adulthood and, by doing so, this pamphlet was the only one to show adults. The photos are more than just a sequence of happy smiling snapshots. Images of children laughing and smiling are very important, but other positive images are also important. The small children in this pamphlet are portrayed engaged in different activities. One is concentrating on painting, another is cleaning her teeth and there is a very tender photo of a girl cradling a doll in her arms. The teenager is in his Boy Scouts uniform, the young male adult is shown vacuuming a floor, and the final image is of an adult working at some kind of machine. These images were, for me, an inspiration, a way forward; they signalled hope.

Without any theoretical analysis, I had instinctively thought that images of Will were crucial to *Will, My Son*. I wanted the reader to carry with them through the text an image of a baby who was, in every sense, a person. As a parent, I was not alone in wishing the world to see and, having seen, to value my child. Other more recent books by parents always include photographs. Indeed, one parent, Charlotte Pelham, has compiled a whole book called *Just Kids* to give a range of images of Down's Syndrome children, showing them in their diversity and capturing their qualities as human beings. It has taken other sectors of society, particularly the charities, much longer to realize and use the importance of positive imagery.

Mencap (The Royal Society for Mentally Handicapped Children and Adults) is the largest charity for people with learning disabilities. Until 1992, its public face, in terms of its 'corporate logo', was that of 'little Stephen' - a line drawing of a sad little boy with tears dropping down his face. In raising the question of the images doctors and parents bring to the moment of disclosure, Dr Bernal handed round the class a number of posters that Mencap had used pre-1992 as part of their fundraising campaigns. The students were asked for their responses and their silence revealed an inability to articulate a response to imagery. Dr Bernal pointed out to them that not one picture showed a child smiling; none of them revealed the subject engaging with life in any meaningful way and, in most, the subjects just looked pathetic. 'I am wondering if those images are the most helpful images to be around when parents are trying to come to terms with the fact that their child has a disability.' One might have asked, too, whether they were the most helpful images for *paediatricians* to hold in their heads.

Aware that their imagery had come under increasing attack from people with learning disabilities, and supported by others, Mencap changed their 'corporate image' in 1992. In their 1992 Annual review, they explained, 'We've dropped our old logo, thought by many to be sad and pathetic, and introduced a new mix of five powerful photographic images to go with the new Mencap logo. The images will appear in print, letters, press and posters nationwide from now on'. So far so good. However, they go on to say, 'The new image is unique and will help our cause to stand out amongst the 150,000 charities in the UK currently competing for resources'. One is left wondering whether or not the motive for changing their imagery was, in fact, primarily one of self-interest. One is also left wondering why the biggest charity claiming to represent people with learning difficulties took so long to think positively. Trying to communicate this positive imagery to the medical profession is, according to their Director of Marketing and Appeals, Steve Billington, not, as yet, on their lobbying agenda.

The Down's Syndrome Association, an organization founded by a parent, Rex Brinkworth, has always realized the importance of positive imagery in its material for members. More recently, they have targeted the general public with positive images and messages designed to change attitudes. One poster of a young, confident girl has the caption, 'Sarah's just learnt to say hello. Can you learn to stop saying Mongol'. Another of a boy about the same age states, 'You say Mongol. We say Down's Syndrome. His mates call him David.' Included in their poster campaign is one that uses the powerful and evocative image of a small, naked baby being held by a young, strong man whose torso is also naked. The caption to this poster reads, 'This child has Down's Syndrome. He also has a future'. At the bottom it adds, 'Having the one child in 660 with Down's Syndrome used to be the end. We've been here for 18 years to make sure it's only the beginning'.

One might wonder whether or not the latter poster is or should be targeted to the medical profession. The Association are, indeed, trying to change images held in the heads of doctors. When I visited St George's Hospital, there was a display mounted by the Down's Syndrome Association in the medical school's library. It was situated near the entrance and covered about four display boards. Besides written information, there were many positive images of Down's Syndrome people, from babies to adults. Dr Bernal urged her students to go and look at the display. If such displays leave only a subliminal impression of a life ahead that involves activity, laughter and relationships, this will still mark a move in the right direction.

Although the charities have taken big steps forward in trying to convey positive images, Britain is far behind the United States in popularizing these images. The American TV series *Life Goes On* which stars Chris Burke, an actor who has Down's Syndrome, is now into its fourth season in the USA. The series is based on the character of Corky, played by Chris Burke. Down's Syndrome, therefore, is central to the stories, but, because it is a series based on Corky and his family, much of it is *also* about a normal family dealing with everyday problems. Sadly, only some ITV companies have chosen to show this series so far. It has won 25 awards in the USA. Even better than just showing an imported series would be if a British TV company were to incorporate a character with Down's Syndrome into a soap or series. British TV soaps and series have lagged far behind the USA in incorporating people with learning difficulties into their cast lists. For the moment, our only screen image of Down's Syndrome is an American series shown only in the daytime in some ITV areas.

One or two of Dr Bernal's students were aware of the series *Life Goes On*. None had actually seen it, though, given its daytime slot, unless they had enough interest to video it and watch it later most, along with others from the medical profession who might benefit from seeing it, go on in ignorance of the achievement of at least one Down's Syndrome person.

There is little evidence that the doctors of the future have a desire to find out more about Down's Syndrome outside of the knowledge they gain from a medical textbook, but the Down's Syndrome Association finds that other health workers often come to them as individuals or as groups to find out more. They told me, 'We often get health visitors, nurses or midwives coming to us for information because they've chosen to do, during their training, a project on Down's Syndrome. But we have just about never had a medical student approach us for more information'. To try and communicate information, besides images, to the medical profession, the Association is planning a conference for community paediatricians and GPs.

Of course, images or even information are no substitute for real knowledge. Real knowledge of Down's Syndrome can only come from direct human contact. For paediatricians seeing Down's Syndrome people only as 'patients', their knowledge is necessarily limited. The change can only come when they, along with other members of the caring professions and the general public, know and accept Down's Syndrome people as part of our everyday life in schools, leisure activities, public places and hospitals. Achieving this will be discussed later in this book.

Although the overwhelming evidence is that paediatricians and parents carry only negative images into the moment of disclosure that a child has learning difficulties, there is always the exception. One of the most extraordinary accounts I have read of such a 'scene' was described by Pat Evans in her article in *The Guardian* (22 December, 1992), 'The best Christmas present of all'. Of the moment of disclosure, Pat Evans wrote, 'The paediatrician arrived, just as we decided to call the baby Euan. He let the baby slip through his fingers, stroking the back of his head with a practised hand. Sitting on the bed he glanced at John, then back at me. "Here comes the tricky bit", he said calmly. "I think your baby's got Down's Syndrome." ' The paediatrician then listed the tell-tale signs and Pat and John responded, like most of us, in stunned, hurt disbelief. The paediatrician continued talking, 'As if his words were a charm to keep our suffering at bay. 'You've ordered from a catalogue and got something back you didn't expect. There is nothing wrong with this baby, he's just different. He's not suffering, you are. He'll be in touch with things we aren't.' He made it sound as if anyone in their right mind would have a Down's Syndrome'. Pat Evans did not immediately accept her paediatrician's view. It took her time to dispel the images of fear and rejection that haunt 'every woman who gives birth to a handicapped child'. In fact, Pat Evans found loving Euan, as I had done Will, 'as natural as falling off a log'. Her article ended with this piece of advice: 'When next you see the parents of a handicapped child, don't automatically feel sorry for them because you have absolutely no idea what they are feeling. Love, in the words of the song, changes everything'.

2 / *What might have been*

Every 14 February I remember Will. It was his birthday. On the 14 February 1993, he would have been 18 – an adult. I wondered what kind of childhood he might have had and what kind of adult life he could kave looked forward to. I have only the experience of others to base my imagination on.

In 1975, I was approached by a producer at the BBC who was interested in making a documentary around a family with a handicapped baby. After discussions between Ed, myself and the producer, we agreed, in principle, to participate.

> The basic structure which the producer suggested and which we agreed to was one based loosely on, or rather inspired by, Humphrey Jenning's *A Diary For Timothy*. It would take this small baby Will as the central person and look at, through us his parents, the kind of life we could expect for our child . . .
>
> The prospect of the film set me thinking, reading and asking questions about the position of handicapped children, the facilities available to them and their parents and of what the future might hold for the handicapped adult. Much that I found out was deeply depressing.

Like the medical profession, my prognosis was based on what had been and what was. Unlike the medical profession, though, I had my hopes and dreams for the future of my child. Those hopes and dreams were not about Will achieving academic or artistic miracles, but were based centrally on the hope that my child would have a place in and be valued by society. In 1975, that seemed a far-off dream, but, since then, much greater progress has been made towards achieving that dream than I could have possibly imagined. There is, of course, still a very long way to go.

One of my problems, as I set out to research this film idea, was that there was virtually nothing I could find to *read* about Down's Syndrome outside of medical information. Getting information, any information, was a major struggle from day one.

> Apart from that one visit from the health visitor, no-one else in that first period, no social worker, doctor, nurse or organization approached us to give us any more information about mongolism or even put us in touch with anyone who might help. The one exception was that the Health Visitor told me that the Royal Society for Mentally Handicapped Children ran a counselling service for parents of handicapped children. I made an appointment to see a counsellor and both of us went. It was a bizarre session. We had a lengthy argument with the counsellor about the importance or otherwise of literacy . . .
>
> A few days later I returned to the National Society for Mentally Handicapped Children and scoured their bookshop for any relevant literature. I found little, but once again nothing that was of any concrete help.

Indeed, I found *not one* book for parents, only pamphlets and articles. Soon after that meeting, I was to find out that people with Down's Syndrome can and do become literate. I was lent an extraordinary and bizarre book, *The World Of Nigel Hunt* (N. Darwin Finalyson). It had been written by a boy with Down's Syndrome. The first breakthrough in finding any useful information was when a friend told me of an organization that had been recently founded by Rex Brinkworth, called the Down's Babies Association (a measure of the changed attitude to the life expectancy of Down's Syndrome people is that the Association, over the 18 years of its existence, has changed its name from Down's Babies, to Down's Children to the Down's Syndrome Association). In 1982, Cliff Cunningham's book, *Down's Syndrome* was published; it was the first book published in the UK on Down's Syndrome specifically for parents.

If the quantity of printed material now available on Down's Syndrome in particular and on people with learning difficulties in general is any indicator of change, then the change has been phenomenal. In researching this book, I strolled into the Mencap bookshop. The whole bookshop was filled with rows and rows of books on people with learning difficulties. Books for parents, health professionals, carers and educators, pamphlets and videos. Books talking about Down's Syndrome babies, children, teenagers and adults. The information I found in 1975 only made passing reference to the Down's Syndrome teenager and barely mentioned the adult. In Mencap's 1993 book catalogue, there are 14 books listed under the specialist category Down's Syndrome. Scanning the individual titles among this wealth of printed material, I could not help but feel amazed at the explosion of information that was unimaginable to me, and I am sure other parents of Down's Syndrome babies, in 1975.

Trying to research the proposed film in 1975, I had tried to get some sense of the social history of Down's Syndrome. I could find out almost nothing but could only assume that, prior to the creation of institutions to which people with mental problems (handicapped and ill) were sent, those that survived must have been cared for in the community. I would have devoured Brian Stratford's book *Down's Syndrome Past, Present and Future,* but it was only published in 1989. The social history that he details confirmed my assumptions. The chapter that particularly caught my attention when I did read it, however, was the one that explores historical attitudes and artistic representations of Down's Syndrome. In it I read that there is a 'healthy discussion' among the experts as to whether or not the sculptures that were done by the Olmecs (people who lived round the Gulf of Mexico some two thousand years ago) are *really* representations of Down's syndrome or whether or not there is some other explanation. However, the information contained in this chapter that most touched me was that, 'There is a painting of the *Madonna and Child* by Mantegna, painted when Mantegna was the court painter for the rich and powerful Gonzaga family in fifteenth-century Mantua. The child is undoubtedly a child with Down's Syndrome'. That there was a time when such a sacred symbol of society, that of the baby Jesus, could have been portrayed as being a Down's Syndrome baby was a revelation to me. It is not because I have Christian beliefs that the image so touches me, because I don't. I am touched by this image of true integration. The nearest modern image of such integration was Mothercare's choosing a young girl with Down's Syndrome to be one of the models for their 1990 catalogue.

Segregation of the mentally handicapped and the mentally ill from society began seriously in the West in the nineteenth century. It became increasingly systematized in the twentieth century, reaching its nadir in fascist Germany where the mentally handicapped were segregated in concentration camps and many were exterminated. For the mentally handicapped in Britain, the twentieth century did bring improved care, but that care was informed by the notion of segregation. This was not changed by the formation of the Welfare State. Indeed, the Welfare State enabled, by means of financial support, the further removal of children from the community who might otherwise, as a result of poverty, have remained within it. I found in 1975 that the future we could expect for Will, based on what was then the case, would be his removal from normal society for education, occupation and possibly even for his daily life.

This last possibility, that Will might or should be put into some form of care, was one I refused to entertain. Ed and I reacted immediately and instinctively to our child.

> At no point did either Ed or I think of rejecting Will. It just did not enter our heads or our hearts. We did not know then that parents could and did sometimes reject their child. We did not know that some people leave their handicapped babies in hospital and leave other people to arrange care. We knew nothing about children who were not normal; nor did we know anything about their parents.

Some other people, however, appeared 'to know' and on the basis of this knowledge gave us advice. They suggested that, in the fullness of time, when he was a little older, maybe as old as a teenager, he and we would be better if he was in some 'home'. This was accompanied by dire warnings that our relationship could not survive the stresses and strains of parenting a child with Down's Syndrome. Even my GP suggested that 'we might well at some stage have to face making a decision between our relationship and our child'. I would listen to these warnings politely, unsure publicly of my new role as the mother of a child with a disability, but inside I would feel like a fiercely protective lioness who was not going to let society get my child.

In assessing for the Portsmouth Down's Syndrome Trust the research done over the last 20 years into the effects on the family of caring for a child with Down's Syndrome, Sue Buckley sums up well the commonly held attitude of the mid-seventies: 'Twenty years ago, the professional view was rather negative. Parents were often advised to put the baby in a home for the sake of themselves and their other children. In other words it was assumed that the effects of bringing up a child with a disability were always negative and that everyone was bound to suffer'. That was certainly an attitude expressed to us and, at the time, I had no way of knowing whether what people were saying to us was true or not.

Research has shown that, once again, there is a wide gap between reality and commonly held attitudes. In his book *Down's Syndrome*, Cliff Cunningham states quite categorically, 'There is no evidence that having a child in the family automatically produces ill-effects in the other children. There is no evidence that couples who have a child with Down's Syndrome are more likely to separate than other couples. In fact there is evidence that many families gain from the experience'. *This* assertion was based on solid evidence.

Cliff Cunningham and his colleagues at the Hester Adrian Centre in Manchester monitored 181 children with Down's Syndrome and their families between 1973 and 1980. Sue Buckley summed up their findings in relation to marital relationships. 'Only 7% of marital relationships in the families with Down's Syndrome were rated as "poor", with 28% being rated as "good" and 65% as "average". This compares very favourably with studies of ordinary families where 22–28% were rated as "poor" or "very poor" '. When asked how they felt their marriages had changed since the birth of their special child, '30% of mothers felt that their relationship with their husbands had improved, 37% reported no change, 15% better in some ways, worse in others, and 14% felt their relationship had deteriorated (4% were single parents)'. Overall, Sue Buckley commented that this study found that, 'Most families were doing fine despite the extra challenges. Those families experiencing greater stress had greater problems than the majority. They had either a child with greater needs, or additional social or emotional stresses to contend with than the families who were doing well. Many of these stresses were not a direct result of having a special child'. American studies have also found that 'Children with Down's Syndrome may have a positive affect on the family climate'.

So, contrary to the received wisdom of the mid-seventies, our relationship would have, in fact, had a slightly better, not worse, chance of survival with Will as part of our family.

Although I instinctively knew that Will's place was in our home, it was only later that I found out that, by the mid-seventies, the emphasis was shifting to encouraging parents to keep their child. The people around us were divided in their attitudes. There had been those friends and professionals who had advised us, for the sake of our well-being, that Will, at some point, should be put in 'a home'. There were also other professionals, relatives and friends who simply supported us in our decision to have Will at home. They supported us not explicitly, but implicitly, by accepting him and us. However, I had no 'role model' of a family with a Down's Syndrome child as its member to look to. I had no concept of it and had trouble imagining how or whether we, myself in particular, could lead a normal life. At least not until we were invited to dinner with a couple who had a teenage Down's Syndrome daughter and two sons.

The experience was like the opening up of a future. I was amazed to find that Molly (Mrs B in *Will, My Son*) 'worked, entertained, went on holidays and led a normal life'. Later, I discussed the 'reality' of that life when, for this book, I went to talk with the eldest son, Colin. During our conversation he commented, wryly, that he was sure his mother presented to us a very positive picture of an integrated family. Very quickly I responded that I was deeply grateful at the time that that was the picture she portrayed to me. It gave me hope. In *Will, My Son* I wrote:

> I left the dinner feeling that for me, as a woman, life could and would go on and that I need not be totally submerged into the small enclosed world of handicap.

For this book, one of the questions I asked Colin was whether or not the break-up of his parents marriage had been 'caused' by the strain of caring for Tessa (called Anna in *Will, My Son*.) His answer was quite categorical, 'I think no matter what children my parents had had they would have broken up. If my sister hadn't been Down's, I think my mother was right, she probably would have left my father a lot sooner. I don't remember them ever being loving with each other. I don't remember them ever being a couple'.

Parents now have many, many more sources to which they can turn for all kinds of information. There is what they see around them, Down's Syndrome children increasingly visible as members of families. There are organizations, particularly the Down's Syndrome Association, as well as other local support groups and organizations to which they can turn. There are also books, some by parents about their own experiences of parenting a child with Down's Syndrome. The most eloquent insight into the world of families, living now with a Down's Syndrome child as a member, is *Living In The Real World*, edited by C. F. Goodey.

The book is constructed from taped interviews with a number of families living in the London Borough of Newham. As would have been expected from the location, the interviewees form a racially mixed group; few consider themselves to be middle class and like any other group of families in 1990s Britain, they are living within a variety of different relationships – married, remarried, single parents and those with partners.

At one level, what emerges from the book is the 'matter of factness' with which the parents speak. For them, having a Down's Syndrome child is a fact of life that they get on and live with. At another level, the book is profoundly moving. It is a testament to the capacity of people for love, care and personal growth. There is no evidence that their relationships have been broken by the strain. Those that were already heading for a break-up, broke up and those that were solidly based remained solidly based.

The other main reason given at the time for, at some point, putting Will in 'a home' was that his presence in the family would be unfair to any other children we might have.

At the time, having another child was not foremost in my mind, but I instinctively thought there had to be another way forward. One way forward has been to recognize the problem, accept it and help siblings and families to work through it. In the late 1980s, Mencap, influenced by organizations abroad, formed a support organization for siblings called SIBS. The recurrent themes that emerge reveal that being a sibling of someone with learning difficulties can be an emotionally difficult and guilt-ridden experience. These feelings are powerfully summed up by a sibling who wrote, 'I am sentenced to guilt, guilt that has haunted me every day since I became of a thinking, and reasoning age. I cannot bring myself to say the words that would give my 80-year-old mother the peace she requires – 'I will give my sister a home for life' – any more than, as a child, I was able to say I would take her with me on social occasions'.

Of course, each family has its own internal dynamics and families are part of society. Both these factors have a profound influence on the siblings. When I thought of the different areas I wanted to explore for this book, one I knew that I wanted to follow up was the family that had invited us to dinner. I had kept in touch with Molly (Mrs B) over the years, mainly through Christmas cards in which we had both enclosed a letter summarizing our previous year's activities. Included, always, in Molly's letter to me was information of Tessa's progress. We had visited her once or twice and had gone to Tessa's eighteenth birthday party. Sadly, I could not talk to Molly for this book; she died in 1992. With my friend, Yvonne Richards, who had first introduced me to Molly, I visited Molly both early in 1992, when she was, we all thought, recovering from an operation for cancer, and, later that year, shortly before she died. I attended her funeral and was amazed at the huge and diverse number of people there. Molly must have touched the lives of many people.

Molly's eldest son, Colin, agreed to talk to me about his experiences and feelings. What emerged from our long conversation was an insight into the pressures that society puts on a family by its attitude to Down's Syndrome. Colin was three when Tessa was born in 1962. His father's immediate reaction to the diagnosis, Colin was told, was 'to phone up the first home to put her away', but his mother would 'not hear of it'. Colin felt his problems, from an early age, were triggered by the attitudes of the time. He felt that his parents, like 'A lot of parents, especially if they decide to keep the child, want to be really, really good about it and say this isn't a special child, they're just like anyone else, they're not different. We are going to treat them just the same. It was, though it wasn't around in those days, a form of political correctness. But for me that skirts around the differences. For me you should acknowledge the differences because difference isn't a bad thing'. Acknowledging the difference was difficult when, publicly, it was not talked about. 'I think the neighbourhood we lived in, being a very middle-class neighbourhood, it was an embarrassment for a lot of people. They couldn't talk about it. They didn't know how to relate to my sister as she got older. When you are surrounded by that attitude; when you also feel that in some way you have failed in producing this child; plus you have then decided to keep it, there is this enormous pressure on you to almost pretend it hasn't happened, which, to me, is quite the wrong thing to do. I think almost the first thing that happened was this conspiracy not to talk about it; not to acknowledge what had happened really; for my parents not to acknowledge that they were really, really upset. I think they didn't want to be upset because to be upset would be to say something was wrong and to say something was wrong was all too horrendous. They clamped down and once you start from that point of view there is often no recovery'.

Because of social prejudice, Colin recognized that his parents were then emotionally forced into a position of defending their child. Their response, he felt, to the knowledge that the world saw Tessa as a 'Mongol', with all the connotations of that word, was to construct the opposite persona, that of an angel. 'You don't want to say that having a Down's Syndrome child is bad or wrong so, therefore, you can't say anything is wrong, so you construct this fantasy of the ideal child, you over egg the pudding wildly'.

Colin's analysis of his parents' reaction to Tessa, his mother's in particular, had deep resonances with my own experience. I *did* acknowledge the difference, though – having Will more than a decade later probably helped in that. However, I also felt fiercely defensive. I remember Colin's mother saying to me as we discussed our feelings for our Down's Syndrome children, 'I know you find your mother love working overtime'. Mine certainly did. For Colin he felt his mother's love worked overtime for Tessa, to the detriment of him and his brother.

The social prejudice Colin keenly sensed as a child and the public pretence of normality was hard to maintain, particularly from the moment Tessa started going to school. 'From a very early age, she was picked up by the school coach. That was a weird thing in the street where I lived. Everyone took their children to school by car, so when this local authority bus, often a coach, would come down the street and would wait outside, it was very unusual. It really marked us out'. Having friends home to play was also something Colin evaded. With hindsight, he feels his evasion was probably for a number of reasons. Partly, it was because of his embarrassment about Tessa, partly, because his mother (for whatever reason) did not encourage him to do so and, partly, because she, through her own disability, which gave her limited mobility, would make Colin do many domestic chores. In front of his friends, who at that period were never to be seen with their hands in the washing-up bowl, he felt deep embarrassment. What went on in the home was almost entirely influenced by his mother. Colin saw little of his father during his childhood, who largely absented himself by working long hours'.

Although living with a Down's Syndrome sister in the sixties was socially embarrassing, it was the problems within the dynamics of the family that caused Colin much more long-lasting psychological problems. Within the family, difference *was* acknowledged, but acknowledged in a way that was not constructive for *any* of the children. Living with an angel was hard on the siblings: 'I remember from a very, very young age being told no matter what you think of what she does, no matter how she behaves you musn't be cross with her. You have to ignore it or forgive her because she can't help it'. This, again, glossed over the differences. 'What happened', Colin explained, 'was that this dynamic was set up with me, less so with my brother because he was younger, that all her naughtinesses were forgiven. That was because if she was being naughty, she wasn't being a naughty girl, she was being a Down's girl. Down's was speaking, not her naughtiness. But children *are* naughty, children play up, children have tantrums, children are loving and it doesn't change because they are Down's. I used to think, even as a child, "But she is just being a pain". For Colin, it both *felt* and *was* unfair. He acknowledges that the same demands could not be made on Tessa as were made on him, but, within the limits of her abilities, demands certainly could, and he felt should, have been made.

Colin felt that he had to become adult and responsible from a very young age. In many ways his childhood was denied him. He also felt he had to hide his own achievements. He lived with a sense of guilt that he had the privilege of being normal and, therefore, could in no way mention, let alone boast about or celebrate, his achievements. So deep was Colin's guilt, he said, 'I was ashamed of what I could do' and, yet, because such pressure was put on him to be adult and responsible, there was another part of him that felt whatever he did was 'not good enough'. As an adult he still carries these two feelings.

For Colin, having a Down's Syndrome sister is a fact of life. He does not see her as an angel, but as a person with a character of her own. Like the relationship between most siblings, he feels a mixture of emotions. His advice to other families with a Down's Syndrome member would be to acknowledge the difference. He knows, from his own feelings for Tessa, that this acknowledgment in no way means you love or care for that person any the less. It goes further. By accepting that she is different, within that difference he can also accept her normality. He doesn't see her as 'Down's' he sees her as his sister, Tessa, whom he knows rather well. One story illustrates this understanding.

After the break-up of his parents, his mother went through a period of deep depression and heavy drinking. Tessa, who was living with her mother, became pitifully thin, almost anorexic. Down's Syndrome people tend to obesity, not anorexia. Because of her extra chromosome, everyone was convinced the cause must be physical, but Colin had no doubt that it was emotional. Like any child, she was expressing her distress at the breaking up of her parents and the obvious, emotional state of her mother. Not eating was, for Tessa, a way of getting attention. Colin admitted that he, as a child, knew that the one way he could get attention from his mother was to be ill. Tessa, he also knew, was not that different from himself.

All siblings can have feelings of rivalry and jealousy – that is normal. The more society can accept that a family with a Down's Syndrome child is normal, the more the family will be able to accept each child as equal, but different. For parents now, the hope is that they do not feel forced into the defensive position that Colin's parents felt they had to take. Sue Buckley, summarizing the research done by the Hester Adrian centre into families with a Down's Syndrome child, found that 'The children and their brothers and sisters had the same range of activities and friendships as other children at the same stage of development. Relationships with brothers and sisters were excellent in most families and there was no evidence that brothers and sisters were more likely to develop behavioural problems than in any other family. 83% of families reported no problems in relationships between the child with Down's Syndrome and their brothers and sisters, 14% some problems and 3% marked problems'. The parents from Newham speaking in *Living In The Real World* give no indication that they feel their other children have in any way been adversely affected by having a brother or sister with Down's Syndrome. Until this generation of siblings grows up and speaks for itself of its experiences, it will be hard to know exactly what they feel. The evidence is that it will have been easier for them than for those, like Colin, who were children in the sixties. As Colin commented, 'the swinging sixties passed us by'. It may have been a decade of liberation for some, but not for the parents or families of children with learning difficulties.

From the evidence of the parents in Newham, things are better in the nineties, but parents still feel the pressure of 'us against the world', or, at least, part of the world. Most had experienced the negativity of the medical profession and some found that their friends and relatives were unsupportive. Few speak of experiencing outright prejudice, though one story reveals that it is still alive and kicking. One mother, a hairdresser, told the interviewer, 'I lost quite a few customers when John was born. They just never came back no more, and if I see them out in the street some would stop and talk, but some never. But out of those few who stayed away, I got the other half who stayed here, and they were really good and that's what I call good friends'. Some of those who had stayed away came dribbling back. When they did she asked them 'But you didn't want to know me at the time, because I had a mongol kid. What's you think, it was catching or something?' Mostly parents felt other people simply did not understand their feelings of love for their child. I could identify absolutely when one father eloquently summed up this lack of understanding by saying, 'I'm proud to have him as my son, I always will be. But, no, I think people sometimes think, well, how can he say that? You can see what they are thinking. "Oh yeah, he's just saying that to put a brave face on it." They don't understand because they've never had the experience'.

EDUCATION

For almost all parents, the way forward to wider social acceptance of their child is through education. Only this kind of contact they feel can break down the barriers of ignorance and fear - barriers many of them recognized as having also been part of their own attitudes until having a Down's Syndrome child had changed them. This attitudinal change is summed up by one father who, in *Living In The Real World*, said, 'But because you've got someone who isn't normal, you know you're thinking, My God, are they going to be part of society? Will society accept them? Because *you* didn't, as a child; you kept saying they're loony, they're not part of society because they're locked away from society, and most people think that when they grow up. But I've got rid of that'. I got rid of it, too, in nine, short months.

For me, like for so many other parents, then and now, integrated education is absolutely central to bringing about greater mutual understanding and acceptance.

As I found out what the situation was actually like for handicapped children and what it could be, were there the political will to change it, I found myself becoming increasingly angry. The thought that my child might be shunted off to a school for the handicapped appalled me.

... It also increased my resolve to fight for the wider changes
needed so that all children could be integrated with the exception
of a very few very severely handicapped.

I wondered, as I set out to write this book, what fights I would
have had and what educational opportunities would have been
offered to Will. To explore this scenario, I went to a friend, Ann
Hollinger, who I knew had both studied and been very involved
in issues related to integrated education.

Ann pointed out that at least Will, born in 1975, was a post the
1971 Act (Education Act – Handicapped Pupils) baby. This Act
had marked a major attitudinal change. It declared that no child
could be deemed ineducable and shifted the care of children
with severe learning difficulties (which Will would have been
deemed to have) from Junior Training Centres run by health
professionals to special schools, which were, increasingly, run by
teachers with a specialist training. The education of children
with learning difficulties was moved from the Department of
Health to the Department of Education. 'He wouldn't have been
very old at all', Ann wryly said, 'When you would have had *nice*
medical ladies telling you 'Don't worry about Will and where he
goes to school, we've got this nice school down the road and we'll
provide him with an education from the age of two until he is
nineteen. Don't worry we'll lay on transport for him, we'll arrange
all his medical treatment needs because we'll have a doctor
regularly visiting, he'll get his speech therapy and his
physiotherapy and all this will be on tap for you in this school.
Don't worry about it'. You might have been told about this when
he was even as young as six months'.

Of course I could have gone 'shopping', as Ann called it, to try
and see whether an ordinary nursery school or playgroup would
have accepted him as a member, but, had I done so, I would have
received no professional back-up. His acceptance in such a
normal environment would have been dependent on the good
will of the group or the school. Choosing this alternative would
have meant that I would have had to make my own arrangements
for speech therapy, physiotherapy and any other special
treatment Will might have needed. One can see why so many

parents opted to follow the advice of the 'nice' ladies.

In those days, medical people were the main determiners of which kind of special school a child should be sent to. Although there were an array of special schools, almost routinely, Down's Syndrome children were sent to schools for children with severe learning difficulties. From 1976, educationalists, wanting more of an input in decision making regarding where children should be sent, established a form of assessment known as special educational procedures. This involved getting reports from a cross-section of professionals who knew your child. Unfortunately, if you disagreed with their assessment of your child, there were no formal, agreed local procedures you could use to challenge it. 'You could', Ann said, 'simply dig your heels in and say, "No, I am not sending him there", and the procedure then was that the Community Paediatrician certified him as suitable only for education in this place. If the Community Paediatrician certified him, you could write to the Secretary of State for education and say I don't like this'. Not surprisingly, during the five or six years these procedures were in force, the Secretary of State received very few of these appeals. I wondered whether or not I might have been one of these few appealing or whether the fight would have been too daunting. 'It did leave families with a sense of some room for manoeuvre', Ann commented, 'though there was this horrible medical authority in the background who could do the certifying'.

Opting out of the special school system and into mainstream schools was not, in the late seventies, an impossibility. Dotted around the country there were individual Down's Syndrome children accepted into mainstream infant and junior schools, but this was always on an individual basis and usually because a persistent parent had found a sympathetic head. No extra practical teaching support or assistance would be given as of right. Any offered would be very informal. At five, had Will gone to some form of mainstream pre-schooling, Ann said another option might well have been presented. 'You would have been shown the school for children with moderate learning difficulties', she explained, 'Partly because he would then be five and eligible for a place, but also because he would have been a bit presentable, having been around in ordinary settings and it would be assumed that he had some sort of social confidence. As long as he could speak or looked as though he might speak pretty soon, then that might have been an option. You would still have got transport and all of that'.

From one pamphlet, *Judith: Teaching Our Mongol Baby* (National Society for Mentally Handicapped Children), which I had acquired while Will was alive, I had been aware that other options were open, and that Down's Syndrome children could achieve more than was generally believed. In this pamphlet, W. W. Smith describes how he and his wife, with some outside help, educated Judith at home until the age of six, when she started attending an educationally subnormal (ESN) school. The pamphlet ends with Mr Smith describing a visit by one of Her Majesty's School Inspectors to the school when Judith was in her seventh year. One can feel the father's pride as he recounts, 'The lady said to Judith's teacher "Oh look at that little one over there pretending to read". They both walked over to Judith who promptly surprised them by reading aloud from the book. The HMI thought it incredible that a six-year-old mongol should be reading such a book, and so well'.

'At the time', Ann Hollinger said, continuing her scenario for Will's educational opportunities, 'You, as a clued-up middle-class parent, would have been very aware that going through Parliament was a new law that, it was said, was going to open up more possibilities for more children with disabilities to go to mainstream schools'. A Royal Commission, chaired by Baroness Warnock, looked into the whole array of special schooling that had grown up since the 1944 Education Act. I had been aware that, in the USA, movement towards integrated schooling was further advanced than in Britain. I wrote in *Will, My Son*:

> The state of Massachusetts pioneered the practical application of the theory that handicapped children should be integrated into the normal state school system. Early experiments were given legal backing in 1974 by a state law, the Bartley Daley Act. The Act marked a great breakthrough. It stopped the categorization of children into normal, sub-normal and severely sub-normal and replaced it with the concept of children with special needs.

The Warnock report, influenced in part by ideas from the USA, was used to frame the legislation carried in 1981. Like the Bartley Daley Act, the 1981 British Education Act required the end of the categorization of children with learning difficulties and, in its place, introduced the overall description of children with 'special educational needs'. To assess each child's individual special educational needs, the assessment process was formalized into what was called the 1981 Assessment and Statement Procedures. This requires, by law, that parents sign their agreement to their child being assessed. It also requires that professionals consult with the family. When this assessment procedure is completed, a formal statement is presented to the parents. This statement is the local authorities' view, based on professional assessment, of your child's special educational needs.

Theoretically, a statement of need should be drawn up for every child with a disability. However, a survey by the Centre for Studies on Integration in Education found in 1993 (ten years after 1983, the year the Act was required to be operational) that, having analysed 15 local education authorities, between 15 and 50 per cent of children in special schools – a total of more than 4000 pupils – were without the protection of a statement of needs. This not only contravenes the 1981 Education Act but also deprives the children of having their special needs identified and provision made for them. It deprives parents of the right to make choices for their child, including the possibility of mainstream education.

Only time will reveal whether or not the new Education Act, due to come into force in 1994, will improve educational choice and opportunities for children with learning difficulties. The Act requires that all schools publish information on how they meet children's special educational needs. Among other changes, the Act will give parents the right to appeal to a tribunal if the local educational authority does not issue a statement of need.

For parents, the process of achieving their right to a statement of their child's special needs means subjecting their child (and they feel themselves, too) to a process of evaluation. Of all the professionals that parents have to deal with, educational psychologists are the most criticized by parents. The parents of

Newham speak almost with one united voice in their criticism of 'the tests' their children are subjected to and 'the testers'. One mother refers to the educational psychologist she had to deal with as 'Miss Plum-in-her-gob'. Need one say more. The parents, however, do say more, and at length. For parents, a huge amount is at stake, especially for those who want their child to go to a mainstream school. For them, going to a mainstream school is the entry point for their child into mainstream *life*.

Understandably, parents feel deep resentment that their child is subjected to 'tests', almost like a laboratory animal. Indeed, the children are tested in, to all intents and purposes, a laboratory. 'I suppose somewhere along the line', one mother said of her son's tests, 'somebody decided that putting three bricks in a little bridge and pushing a pencil through indicates some skill or other, but I've never really understood how relevant it was to Richard. I used to think it must be very important that he won't play with these bricks because she used to do a lot of writing at that point. But if a child doesn't like playing with bricks, I don't see how you can judge what mental age they're at simply because they don't like playing with them'. Whether it was bricks, puzzles or other forms of IQ testing, all the parents interviewed in Newham thought them inappropriate tests. Time and time again, the parents complained that their knowledge of their child's abilities and limitations was not considered as valid evidence. One parent summed up the situation succinctly: 'I could never understand what their aims were when they said, you know, we've all got the same aims in common. They know better. They wanted one thing, we wanted another. It's never been an equal partnership. They say it is, but, of course, it ain't. How can it be an equal partnership when they have little caucus meetings on their own? There's never been equal partnership going on, and there never will be. Because professionals don't think parents *are* equal'. Parents of whatever class are never equal, but those who are middle class, particularly, if they themselves are health professionals, do get less condescending treatment.

Almost all complain that the professionals have preconceived ideas about their child. As one parent said of his daughter, 'She can't be a person first'. In educational terms, this means that they 'measure' the child in terms of preconceived ideas about what a Down's Syndrome child can and can't achieve, with the emphasis being largely on the latter. For them, achievement is in conventional terms. The parents have a much wider definition of achievement. What is interesting is that the parents are both very realistic about their own children's abilities – whether it be dressing themselves, kicking a football, eating in a socially acceptable manner or reading – and much more open about their children's potentialities. While having their feet firmly rooted to the ground, they also see the sky as the only limit.

The complaint by parents that professionals see their children as Down's Syndrome, not as people, is almost universal. This applies to all aspects of the children's lives – their abilities, health and psychological problems. Those that know them as a person, just as Colin knows his sister Tessa, *respond* to them as a person.

Finding understanding of this by the professionals can be hard. Lucy Baxter, after adopting James, found out that his early childhood had been one of neglect and abuse. Had James been a normal child, his psychological problems would have been recognized and he would have been offered therapy, but health professionals, educationalists and psychologists see him only as Down's Syndrome; the definition of handicap overrules looking at a child as an individual. Those who *know* children with Down's Syndrome are aware that their differences are greater than their similarities because they know them as people first. Ignorance is to be found in all spheres of life. I was staggered when a vicar's wife, a sort of professional in my mind, said to me after Molly's funeral that she couldn't understand why they had brought Tessa to the funeral. All I could reply was 'Most of us find it pretty hard to comprehend death. Funeral's sort of help'. I wondered what preconceived idea she had of Down's Syndrome.

In pursuing a mainstream school place for Will, I could see it would have involved a struggle – probably a fight. I asked Ann whether or not, for me, as a parent of a six-year-old Down's Syndrome child in 1981, the Act would have enabled me to say, 'My child has a right to go to a mainstream school'? The answer, like the wording of the Act, was not a simple 'yes' or 'no'. There were those parents, supported by people like Ann, who campaigned for this right. They were the people who wanted to put the 'yes' potential of the Act to the test. The campaigners found that, when faced with the reality of the provisions made by local educational authorities, no such right existed in practice. One of the problems was that each local educational authority had developed its own array of special schools over the years and each local authority had to review its provisions, some with more commitment to achieving integration than others. This commitment, if it came, was often a result of political pressure put on the local authority by local campaigning groups.

An analysis of how the London borough of Newham came to adopt a 'Statement of Intent' to desegregate its schools in 1987 was published in 1991 (London Borough's Disability Resource Team), entitled *Newham Makes Integration Work*. This analysis, carried out by the London borough's Disability Resource Team, provides an insight into the attitudes held by different sectors of the community to the issue. These attitudes are to be found in every local authority, but what differs is which power group wins out. In Newham, from the outset, there was a clash. The local authority, including its education officers, felt that only a little tinkering needed to be done to their system of education to comply with the requirements of the Act. Parents of children with disabilities thought otherwise. They saw the Act as a means of enabling radical change. The Schools Sub-Committee, responding to the views of the parents, set up a Working Party to draft a policy document. The Working Party, comprised of parents, teachers and councillors, found that, when the time came for making their recommendations, they were divided: 'Some members were arguing that separate special schools were the natural setting for education of children with learning and other disabilities. The rest were asserting that such segregation was both morally and educationally indefensible'. For a year, the matter remained unresolved. During this time, each side of the debate mustered support for their arguments and each side lobbied their councillors. In the middle of this debate, 1986, the local elections took place and the Newham Labour Party group made a manifesto commitment to furthering integration. With integration as a political priority, the Labour Party, having been returned to power there, soon became committed to making an immediate start to planning for integration. Having won the moral argument, for Newham, as for other boroughs it then becomes a practical problem of planning and the transferring of resources to make integration meaningful.

The authors of the report, in analysing 'what tipped the balance', concluded that several factors had come into play. However, the factor that they found had been paramount in tipping the balance was the 'users of special educational services'. They spearheaded the pressure for change, and 'Local politicians created opportunities for debate about possible directions for change, and actual choices were made under the direction of dedicated individuals committed to securing equality within the education system for young people with disabilities and learning and other significant difficulties'. It was because of these 'users', supported by others, that this report could open with the words, 'A quiet revolution is underway in the London borough of Newham. Special educational provision is being progressively desegregated'.

This 'quiet revolution' is not happening in all local authorities. The forces *against* radical change have the power in many of them. Local councillors and education officers who feel little change is needed are often supported by some parents as they were in Newham. Integration is not necessarily welcomed by all parents. When the then Inner London Education Authority made public its report outlining its proposals for the phased introduction of integration, which would involve the moving of resources over time from special schools to mainstream schools, many parents protested. Some parents protested and demonstrated with banners saying 'Save our special schools'. These parents, like others, feel that special schools provide a safe and protective environment for their children. They also protect the parent from having to deal with the prejudice of society. Their position is supported by an educational position that argues that children can better learn skills in a safe, protected environment that they can then take out into the world. The special schools themselves also, obviously, have an interest to protect. These parents supporting the continued existence of special schools are mainly parents whose children were or are already in these schools.

Parents now facing the question of what kind of education to choose for their Down's Syndrome child wish their child to be integrated into a mainstream school. The Down's Syndrome Association finds that almost all their parents want mainstream schooling for their child and almost all parents have to fight for it. One father from Newham expressed what most parents think: 'It should be made available, there shouldn't be any question of it – they shouldn't *have* to go to special schools. If a child needs help, he should get it'. Unfortunately, many parents face a large number of obstacles in trying to get their child into a mainstream school and, once there, in getting the help and resources their child needs within that school. Various bodies offer independent advice and help to parents. The fact that charities, such as the Independent Panel for Special Education Advice, have had to be set up to help parents get what should be their right is a reflection of the low commitment of most educational authorities to integrated schooling. All too often, statements are drawn up that fit the child into what is available rather than, say, what the child really needs.

Mainstream schools may believe in integrated schooling in theory, but, in practice, are reluctant to take in children with disabilities unless resources and funding have been transferred to them or are guaranteed. The business of changing the educational system to one that is based on integration obviously could not happen overnight. However, the speed of change is very variable from local authority to local authority. So, from 1983, although you could demand to have your child accepted into a mainstream school, there was no guarantee that this demand would be met. If Will had fallen into the average to brighter group of Down's Syndrome children, there would have been a reasonable chance of getting him into a mainstream school at the junior level. In general, at the infant and junior school levels, integration is progressing, with many more schools accepting children with disabilities, particularly if the funding for trained back-up is made available.

I then asked Ann what would have happened when Will was

11. 'Well, there is *the gap* you know', Ann replied. I asked 'What is the gap?' 'Well', she said, imitating the arguments, 'it is all right for these children at infant and junior level, they can muck in and get by, but, as they get older, the gap between them and their peers increases in unmanageable ways. It is just not good for them to be unable to grasp what goes on in secondary schools. It is not fair to the child.' Our best option, Ann thought, would probably have been to move from Brent, where we were living, to another local educational authority that had transferred resources to mainstream schools so that children with disabilities could be admitted, supported and the child's special needs catered for. The provision of such resourced secondary schools varies enormously from one authority to another. Parents can and do move house to get the kind of education they want for their child.

All this, however, has marked a major change since 1975. This change is summed up by quoting from two pamphlets. *Your Mongol Baby*, published by MIND, that I obtained in the seventies, tried to reassure me as the parent of a newborn Down's Syndrome baby that, in terms of education, 'All children are legally entitled to appropriate education from the age of five years and special schools are provided in every local education authority. They cater for children whose abilities are limited and who, therefore, need particular understanding and teaching methods adapted to their needs'. A new parent can now receive a pamphlet from the Down's Syndrome Association called *Your Questions Answered*, which states that 'People with Down's Syndrome can learn effectively. They are described however as having "special educational needs" and will therefore require special educational provision. The trend following the 1981 Education Act has been towards integration of children with Down's Syndrome into "ordinary schools" rather than segregation in "special schools" '. The change goes even further. Glancing along the rows of books relating to the education of children with learning difficulties, my eye stopped at one the title of which was *Literacy For All* and its subtitle explained *A whole language approach to the English National Curriculum for pupils with severe and complex learning difficulties*. For me, the title was striking because it symbolized a commitment to integration, a commitment to accepting children with learning difficulties into mainstream education. The fact that the 1988 Education Act states that all children have an entitlement to a broad and balanced curriculum as its main aim and that any modification or disapplication of this clause has to be agreed, changes the balance of rights.

Although the practice falls far short of the entitlement, what has changed since 1975 is that asking that one's Down's Syndrome child be accepted into a mainstream school has become a legitimate demand. Behind this demand, however, is much, much more. It was felt that, in the past, special schools had low expectations of children with Down's Syndrome, and children have a habit of achieving what is expected of them. Going to a mainstream school is a way of allowing the child with Down's Syndrome to maximize their potential. Instead of saying 'your child will not achieve anything', those involved are saying, implicitly, there are many things your child will achieve, but, as your child is an individual, we do not know exactly where their talents will lie. Integrated education allows the Down's Syndrome child a chance to be part of the community. It also allows the community to learn about children with Down's Syndrome. Integration is about the education of our society as a two-way process. For parents with the hope that their child will grow up as part of and be accepted by the community, integrated education is absolutely central. It is hardly surprising that they feel so much is at stake when their child is assessed. Unfortunately, parents are in the hands of assessors who did not have the benefit of integrated education. Of them, one father in Newham commented, 'As far as I am concerned, I think the professionals are the ones who need sorting out . . . they haven't got any comprehension, because they see things like – *that* [puts his hands to the sides of his face like blinkers]. Let's face it, it was experts who used to say the Earth was flat, so you can always change your mind. The question is, who assesses the assessors?' The blinkers are still on most professionals, but the parents are fighting and adult Down's Syndrome people are proving them wrong.

ADULT LIFE

What Will's future as an adult would be was something that concerned me from the moment I was told he had Down's Syndrome. My first question had been, 'What will happen to him when he grows up?' My first reaction was to see 'the rest of my life mapped out – a life inextricably linked to my handicapped child'. Feeling overwhelmed by the future is a common reaction of parents on first learning about their child's disability. Later, in thinking of his future:

> I feared for what would happen to him if we died before him; I feared for how I would cope with having an adult dependent on me for the rest of my life; I feared for how society would treat him as an adult. Whilst people are usually sympathetic towards a handicapped child, sympathy is absent in most people's treatment of handicapped adults. The options for a handicapped adult who cannot live an independent life are bleak and equally bleak are the options for the responsible relatives.

Had Will lived, his options in 1993 would have been much greater than any I could have envisaged back then. Part of my problem in picturing any options was that few were presented to me. The literature I had talked almost exclusively about children's early years. Those that projected forward painted such a depressing picture that I recoiled with horror. The MIND pamphlet informed me that, 'At the age of 16, most mongol children will have progressed from the spontaneous activities of the nursery group to be ready for transfer to an adult training centre'. There, the reader is reassured, 'Your child will probably be taught how to handle money, how to use the public telephone and public transport, how to recognise notices such as *danger, open, closed, wait, cross* – in short, how to go about as independently as he can'. There was a ray of hope in the phrase, 'some mongol boys and girls may be found full employment in the community', but this is quickly undercut by the reality that 'most, however, will remain in sheltered workshops'.

Had Will lived, at 16 he would have had a number of options for furthering his education at least until the age of 19. Many of these opportunities are not in segregated schools but in local colleges of further education, some in integrated classes and some in classes for those with learning difficulties. Slowly, educational opportunities are opening up for people with learning difficulties over the age of 19, but, as yet, they are few and far between. In describing the kind of courses available for Down's Syndrome Children over the age of 16, the Down's Syndrome Association lists, among the special courses that may be available, courses in 'personal relationships, sex education and leisure activities'. The inclusion of sex education marks a major attitudinal change. In *Will, My Son* I wrote:

> In my searches there was one question I didn't, or dared not, ask because I was frightened of the reply. It had saddened me to think that Will might grow up denied the possibility of a loving sexual relationship with another person. To talk about the sexual desires and needs of a mentally handicapped adult is to touch upon a very sensitive subject - almost a taboo.

This taboo has been broken. Some people do now recognize that people with a range of disabilities have sexual desires and needs just like everyone else. The Down's Syndrome Association publishes a small leaflet entitled *Sexuality and Down's Syndrome*. Its final statement asserts that 'Given the right education and guidance there is no reason why people with Down's Syndrome should not derive pleasure from sexual relationships at varying levels throughout their lives'. Such a statement marks an enormous change from 1975 when the subject was simply not mentioned.

Sex education in our society is and always has been a contentious issue. The present Conservative Government has shown only a limited commitment to sex education in schools and recent changes to the law will allow parents to withdraw their children from sex education classes. The question of sex education is surrounded with ambivalence, embarrassment and even hostility. Giving sex education to people with learning difficulties, however, touches not just on a question of sexual morality, it touches on the question of the rights of people with learning difficulties to be human beings in every sense of the word. This includes both the right to have sexual relations and the right to reproduce.

The parents speaking in *Living In The Real World* both recognized their children's sexuality, or potential sexuality, and found it perfectly normal. One succinct statement by a parent echoes the thoughts of all of them: 'He'd be fulfilling his life. I sort of treat him as a normal kid, you know'. Because of their child's learning difficulty, parents have heightened worries that their child might be sexually abused or exploited. In the main, however, their worries are the worries of all parents about their children having safe sex and of finding a loving relationship. Their view, they are well aware, is by no means supported by others they know.

The argument for recognition of their children's sexuality goes further than just recognition of a physical need: 'The idea some people have, I think - I've never heard it said outright - is obscene, that they shouldn't be allowed to do it, and that's the clearest way of saying they're not human beings', stated one mother, and she went on to criticize what she saw as another obscenity - the argument about the consequences of Down's Syndrome people having sexual relationships. Her reply was, 'I mean, why is it unfair to let a Down's child be born to a Down's parent when one in however many it is are born to parents who are *not* Down's? I suppose you can say it isn't fair to the child who may not have Down's Syndrome because the parent does have it - well, what children need is to be loved, and I think that's been proved, and there is no reason that a Down's Syndrome mother or father couldn't love their children'. It is hardly surprising to find that none of them saw the sterilization of their child as an acceptable option. The optimism of these parents that their child might find some loving relationship was in stark contrast to my assumption, that although I hoped he might, 'the reality was that it was very unlikely'.

Accepting that people with learning difficulties have a right to sexual expression is the first step. Acceptance of that right is by no means universal among those who care for them. Privacy is a precondition for socially acceptable sex. Many who live in hostels are not allowed locks on their doors. Many living at home find any sexual activity is made equally unacceptable. Because society has not accepted that people with learning difficulties have a right to sexual expression, they have denied these people education about and the opportunity for it. Even parents who believe that their child has a right to sexual expression may find it difficult to talk with and help their child to achieve it. The evidence is that parents find talking to their children about sex difficult and a large number duck out of doing it. If most normal children need sex education from trained people, then the child with learning difficulties has even greater need.

There are books available, organizations and classes for those who accept that there is a need. Colin told me of how the subject of Tessa's sexuality was finally discussed through the agency of a third party. His family, in that respect, is probably little different from many others. Like most families, Colin's did not talk about sexual behaviour, least of all Tessa's. Tessa had learned, through assimilation, what was acceptable public and private behaviour. Colin had only become aware of her 'private' behaviour, masturbation, because Tessa did not have a lock on her room. The subject of Tessa's sexuality was only raised when Molly was invited to Tessa's Day Centre to join in sessions designed to discuss issues of sexuality and she asked if Colin would accompany her. The request for his company he saw as an acknowledgment by his mother of his role in relation to his sister.

Colin felt that the sessions were helpful to many parents in both opening up the issue in the first place and then in giving guidance as to how they could help, educate and respect their child's sexuality. It was interesting that Colin discussed with his mother his sister's sexuality before he could 'come out' and discuss with her his own homosexuality.

Sadly, though, hostility to the rights of people with learning difficulties to sexual expression is still very great. The organization, Young People First, have found that among young adults with learning difficulties, there is great ignorance about their bodies and about sex. One of the educational objectives of Young People First is sex education for these young adults.

Examples of people with Down's Syndrome who were

employed were few and far between in 1975. I did not research
the employment possibilities in any systematic way – that lay too
far ahead – but I clung on to every scrap of information given to
me that signalled this might be a possibility. Before leaving the
hospital in which Will had been born, the Sister of the neonatal
intensive care unit:

> Told me the story of a Down's Syndrome man she had known who
> had worked in a hospital laboratory. She remembered him well
> and described him in great detail. I remembered because it was the
> first example I had heard of a Down's Syndrome adult doing a
> normal job.

This story was so much more positive than the paediatrician's
response about 'sheltered workshops and things being better',
but, then, the Sister, in all her dealings with Will and with me, was
more positive in every way. After that first story, I heard of others,
but they were always individual; the general attitude was that
gainful employment was not on the agenda.

The world of employment is still one in which it is difficult for
Down's Syndrome adults to find a place. Although many have the
skills and abilities required for certain jobs, their chances of
finding employment are slim while unemployment is high and
the economy is in recession. Even when the economic climate is
good, people with learning difficulties face prejudice and
ignorance when seeking employment. Job advertisements may
state that they do not discriminate against people with
disabilities, but, in practice, they do. This discrimination starts
with the charities. Historically, charities themselves have not
employed the people they represent. It is only very recently that
they have been embarrassed into practising what they preach.
For 30 years the law has required that a percentage of people with
disabilities are employed. Only a small number of companies
covered by the law actually employ the 3 per cent quota and the
government has very rarely prosecuted any company for not
complying. Despite prejudice and the economic climate,
though, some Down's Syndrome people do find jobs. The
assumption that a sheltered workshop is the only form of

employment that can be expected for all but the exceptional high-flyer is no longer held by those who know of their capabilities.

In 1992, Mencap, as part of their new image, issued six manifestos to state clearly their intent and direction. These manifestos cover the key issues relating to citizenship, leisure, family life, education, housing and employment. Their manifesto on employment opens by asserting what is true for everyone, 'that having a job is a badge of citizenship'. For people with learning difficulties, having a job shows, Mencap asserts, 'in the clearest possible way their contribution has value. Not only that, the money will open other doors – to getting a home, enjoying leisure, having choice. Employment is the linchpin of personal life'.

In my wildest dreams I did not envisage a future for Will that might be one of self-supporting independence. In 1975, my mother gave me a copy of *The Countryman* in which there was an article about an organization called CARE (Cottage and Rural Enterprises). They had set up a farm village in which people with learning difficulties were living and working. This 'village' was a self-supporting community where, with some supportive help, the disabled members lived and worked. Such communities, at the time, I felt was the most I could aspire to for Will. The other options that I was aware of appalled me. As this article pointed out, 'There are 250 000 mentally handicapped people, of whom 64 000 are adults in mental hospitals, 40 000 needing no treatment but with nowhere else to go. Another 186 000 live at home and are cared for by relatives, or the local authorities give day care'.

The option of a mental hospital was unthinkable. Thinkable, but overwhelming, was the prospect that, for the rest of our lives, we would have a dependant child living with us. Indeed, 60 000 adults with severe learning difficulties do still live with their parents. Many of the parents are now elderly, looking after their adult children of 50 or 60. The parents worry, like all parents whose child has not moved out of home or achieved any independence, supported or otherwise, 'What will happen when I die?'

Theoretically, the 1990 National Health Service and Community Care Act should change all this. It gives people with learning difficulties the right to live in the community and to be offered as much or as little support as they individually need. The theory, indeed the legislation, marks a great leap forward, but the practice has made many question the motives of the Conservative Government who brought in the legislation. Care In The Community can only work when it is well thought through and properly resourced. All too often, local authorities, starved of money directly by the government or because of their own political policies, do not provide the back-up to make care in the community the leap forward it should be. It is not just the Conservative Government whose commitment to genuine Care In The Community can be questioned. Sadly, too often, local communities themselves do not want people with disabilities living in their midst. It seems that there is no better way of bringing people's ignorance, fear and prejudice out into the open than to inform them that some form of housing for people with learning disabilities is to be opened in their street.

The Down's Syndrome Association state in their pamphlet *Your Questions Answered*, 'People with Down's Syndrome will move away from their family home, either when they reach adulthood and feel ready, as with other young people, or when their family is unable to care for them any more. They will generally require some form of supported accommodation'. The thought that Will might, as a young adult, leave home and live in some form of sheltered housing, perhaps sharing a flat with someone else with a warden to hand was not available to me in 1975. Even more unimaginable was that he should live in his own accommodation as a self-supporting adult. Some people with Down's Syndrome do.

The possibility that Will might demand to leave home at some point, equally, never entered my head, until talking to Ann Hollinger. At the end of my discussion with her, when we were discussing the kinds of courses or vocational training that colleges of further education offer she commented, 'Will, of course, would probably be having a wonderful time getting himself involved in self-advocacy groups in his college. He might even join People First, which is a group of young people with learning difficulties who go around talking about their right to choose, their right to make mistakes. They go on about 'Your dreadful parents who do nothing but want to protect you. Here you are at 25 and you still have to ask if you can have a key to go out'. He would probably be into all of that?

On the train going home from seeing Ann, I smiled inwardly to myself at the thought that Will and I might have been battling over his right to independence. It was, of all the changes I found out about, the one that most touched me. It symbolized the emergence of the self-hood of people with learning disabilities; becoming a voice in society is to become a part of society. I am sure I would have been an overprotective parent, terrified about what might happen to my child if I let him out, unprotected, into the world. Although I knew that I wanted my child to have every opportunity to take part in society as a valued member, letting him do so would have been difficult for me. Hopefully, I would have found support in this process, and he would, like my daughter, Jessie, have forced the issue.

3 / Change

THE LANGUAGE OF CHANGE

Both of us felt very strongly that we wanted to make a statement about his life, about our feelings about his life and by implication our feelings about his death. We suspected that many people thought that because he was a Down's Syndrome child, because he was 'different', our feelings might be different. We also suspected that many people would be thinking 'it's really for the best'. Later we didn't even have to suspect that that was what people were thinking, some told us so. The measure of his life was that those people who had known him well grieved with us, we felt, with no reservation. He had changed us and them.

It was at Will's funeral that we wanted to make this statement. Through the words said by a friend, our feelings were made clear. In nine months, Will changed me in a profound way. Prior to his birth, I probably would not have expressed outright prejudice to the 'mentally handicapped', but I certainly saw them as people who were 'not quite human'. I would pity them and their parents. If asked, no doubt I would have said that I was grateful that other members of society - dedicated, professionals - ensured that their basic needs were cared for. I would have been shocked if the press revealed that such people were being treated badly or were living in inhumane conditions, but I would never have questioned that 'they' should be cared for separate from society. I never questioned that this separation in itself was inhumane. People who, to me, looked odd, behaved in funny ways and/or who made inarticulate noises were frightening. I did not know how to behave around them, let alone communicate with them. Then, ten days after Will was born, I found out that my beautiful baby was one of 'them'.

From the outset I never could see him as 'one of them' only as my baby, a human being. I also felt from the outset that he had his own distinctive personality that, as he grew older, became more and more evident.

> As he developed, his human responsiveness and warmth were very evident. They were also very endearing. We, the doting parents, were not the only people to come under this particular form of his charm.

His distinctive personality is also something, besides us, that others have told me they remember. Not long ago, I found myself sitting in a wine bar in Camden with a woman producer who, with her husband, had invited Ed, myself and Will to dinner. I had not met her for years. As we sat sipping wine, talking about business, our families and the struggle to give up smoking, her memories of Will cut through the conversation. She remembered him vividly, his bright face watching everyone and then suddenly cracking up into a huge smile, and, as I listened to her description, I felt both huge pride in him and my deep pain.

One of the things I used to do with Will to entertain him was to put on some music and dance with him in my arms. There was one song we danced to time and time again, a Fats Domino number, *It keeps rainin'*. I would rock him slowly to the rhythm of the music and, then, at the chorus, I would suddenly change the rhythm of the rocking to double speed and whirl him around. He loved it, bursting into gurgles of joy every time. Like his gurgles, the words of the first line of the chorus 'You left me reelin'' and rockin' still echo in my head. They echo not just as a memory, but because they sum up how I look back on that year, 1975. It was as though an emotional wind storm hit, picked me up, threw me around, turned me upside down and then dropped me. I was left, in every way, 'reelin' and rockin''.

One of the parts of me that had been totally rocked was my attitude to people with disabilities. The experience of my son, Will, profoundly changed my attitude to every other son or daughter that I had previously seen as 'them'. They were, after all, other people's sons and daughters. For me, 'they' became part of 'us', part of the human race, part of the diversity that is the human race, but I have moved even further. I recognize that this sentence is patronizing. It is as though 'I' am accepting 'them'. The fact that, as a so-called normal person, I can make this statement is a reflection of power relationships within society. For example, as a woman, a member of the 'weaker sex', I know only too well how men have and do 'so graciously' say we will accept you into our club, place of work, bar, democracy, but not, so far, into the Long Room at Lords.

My mental attitudinal change happened fast and traumatically, but it did not suddenly provide me with information about and understanding of all disabilities. Having Will did not provide me with the knowledge of how to communicate, say, with someone who is deaf. However, it did provide me with the understanding that communication, in whatever form, is something we have to learn. Learning to accept one difference almost certainly predisposes one to accepting another, but it does not provide instant understanding of these other differences. Colin, for whom Down's Syndrome had been part of his normality, found the same: 'For me it is so normal. Tessa was so much part of my life that I forget how, for people who haven't had that proximity – it is like being gay, you see it all the time – I forget how deep those hatreds and prejudices and fears run in people. To me it is normal. She was normal. She was just there. It was not a case of "Oh my God, what am I going to do?", so it is easy to forget that. I forget it, not because I am such a wonderful person but just because of sheer experience. That was how it was. If I hadn't had that I would probably be just the same as other people. I did learn a lesson when I went to university. Although I was very familiar with my sister, other disabilities panicked me, particularly physical ones, people who were in wheelchairs or who were blind or deaf. I assumed I would know how to be. I think I was better, but I still felt I didn't know what I was doing'.

My response to Colin was that such interactions are about progressing 'on a learning curve'. For me, before Will's birth, I hd not even realized that this was what I needed to do. We are not born with a knowledge of the needs of others; we have to learn about them. I admitted that I still could feel inadequate and uncomfortable around people with certain disabilities. Colin agreed, commenting that he gets 'Very cross with some of the politically correct terminology around disability'. Of my feelings of inadequacy he said, 'If you feel like that it is a natural thing. You shouldn't feel bad because you feel inadequate. When people try and put this on to you, that somehow you should know, somehow there is some book of knowledge that the enlightened person knows about and has access to, and if you don't you are somehow a fascist, it is ridiculous. It is absolutely ridiculous. It is a way of thinking I would never get into. If I see somebody going up behaving really strangely with my sister, I'll notice it and think "here we go again", but I won't necessarily think the worse of them. If they keep doing it and never learn, then I'll get cross, but, if it is the first time, or the first few times, how do they know? They are trying it out. You have to let people make mistakes. Obviously, if you are a disabled person, you get really fed up with it and you snap from time to time. Just as people say the most stupid things to me about my sexuality, but I don't always say something. I want people to have the freedom to make mistakes. I wasn't given that freedom in my family and that was a big mistake. My sister was set up as this porcelain, fragile, untouchable figure, which she wasn't. She was this robust, healthy-madam sometimes. It meant we never had a normal relationship'.

Achieving normal relationships between people with differences is the goal of those who have and do campaign for change. Looking at the changes since 1975, it is interesting to see who has spearheaded this change. Where did the understanding, the desire, the energy, the will to effect change spring from?

To look at the change, though, we have, first, to look at what we are changing from. In the western world, white, normal, heterosexual men were the definition of what it is to be a human being. Within that definition the rich, educated and powerful were seen as more 'normal'; everybody else was, in some way other, different, not normal. Over the years all those 'other' groups have fought, and are still fighting, to become accepted as part of normality, to be seen as equal but different. Women, non-white people, the poor, gays, lesbians and people with disabilities all have their struggles.

In these struggles, all have felt that, to bring about new definitions of themselves, they have to change the language that defines them. I quickly changed my language when I learned how and why the term 'mongol' had been used to define this group of people. Long before it was discovered that Down's Syndrome is caused by the existence of an extra chromosome, doctors attempted not only to describe the condition in medical terms but also to attach to this description a theory of its cause. Thus, in the nineteenth century, there were many who believed that *degeneracy* caused the birth of children with learning difficulties. R. Chambers, an exponent of the degeneracy theory, in his book *The Vestiges of the Natural History of Creation*, published in 1844, went further. For him, degeneracy was not just a case of *individual* behaviour it was *racial*: he confidently asserted that 'The Mongolian, Malay, American and Negro, comprehending perhaps five-sixths of mankind, are degenerate'.

John Langdon Down was the first person to study and describe, with care, a group of patients he called 'Mongolian'. This group, with certain common features, were included as one of five groups of patients he described in a paper published in 1866, called 'Observations on an ethnic classification of idiots'. Down's Syndrome thus stems from the work of John Langdon Down, the first physician to recognize that there is a definable group of people with certain characteristics. Sadly, John Langdon Down's description 'Mongolian', with all its racist connotations, was the one that stuck. Almost a century and a half later, people are still trying to un-stick the label.

'Idiots', 'imbeciles', 'lunatics', 'the feeble-minded', 'cretins', 'the mad', 'vegetables' and 'mongols' are just some of the words that were used to describe people with either learning difficulties or mental illness – little distinction was made between the two. These terms now shock us when we read them. As they were dropped from use by those who saw them as offensive, new terminology came into being. Terms such as 'mentally handicapped', 'subnormal' and 'retarded' became the dominant descriptions. All these descriptions were made by one set of people about another, the latter having no say in the matter.

Change has come, however. People with learning difficulties have spoken out and said how they themselves would like to be described. The terms 'learning difficulties' or 'learning disabilities' are *their* choice.

Language does not exist in a vacuum; there is a speaker and one spoken to. I remember chatting away to Will happily and, when he had done something stupid, I would say 'You idiot'. One time, it suddenly struck me that I *could* call him that. For me, he was normal and I could use my normal language to him. If another had said it to him, unless I had felt absolute confidence of the normality of their relationship with him, I would have felt the historic connotations of all that this description of him entailed. I would not have liked it.

Changing language is crucial. Language reflects our feelings and our attitudes. It is an outward and visible symbol. Making someone call the girl in the picture Down's Syndrome, not mongol, does not change their attitudes, but it does change the public expression of an attitude. Speaking of people with respect is a major step in moving towards respecting them. Sadly, the media, far from being leaders in this or any another campaign to change language, lags behind.

The Down's Syndrome Association now issues a brief information sheet for journalists. It explains that, 'Like parents the world over, members of the Down's Syndrome Association think of their children as people first. That is what we want your readers to realise'. In trying to overcome ignorance and prejudice, the Association wants to stress, 'how much we have in common with every other family rather than setting ourselves apart with "tragic" or "heroic" portrayals'. They ask journalists to 'Check their story - is it patronizing, or does it make the person with Down's Syndrome an object of pity? Check your language - avoid describing people with Down's Syndrome as "victim of" or "suffering from". Instead use the phrase "someone who has" or "a person with" '. As I read these guidelines, it took me back to all the campaigns we had had in the 1970s to get the union I belong to, which represents people working in film and television, to draw up a code of conduct relating to sexist language.

We as women had, and still have, good reason for campaigning for a change in the language used by the media to describe us. People with learning difficulties have equal cause for complaint. For six weeks - 15 March to 30 April 1987 - Alison Wertheimer studied press reporting of people with learning difficulties. Her study and analysis, *According to the Papers: Press reporting on people with learning difficulties*, was backed and published by CMH (now called Values Into Action). It was undertaken to try to achieve a better understanding of the opinions held by people about those with learning difficulties. Research has shown that, although many people do know someone with a learning difficulty, it is often the case that an *image* of what *'they'* are like overrules their *personal knowledge* of what an *individual* is like. The individual is usually seen as, in some way, exceptional, not typical. The aim of the study, therefore, was to find out how much the press contributed to the creation and persistence of stereotyped images.

Two major stories broke during that period. One was about the Royal Family. On 6 April 1987, *The Sun* revealed that two first cousins of the Queen had been admitted to the Royal Earlswood Hospital in 1941. One had died there in 1986 and one was still alive. Although the story triggered many headlines and column inches, it did not lead to a public debate about the issues. In contrast, the other big story that broke provoked extensive public debate. Thus, it was of much greater interest in terms of revealing what the press' attitudes were through the language they used. The story was about the case of Jeanette - a pseudonym used to protect her identity. Jeanette was a young woman with learning difficulties who had been in the care of the local authority since she was four. When she was 17, the local authority and her mother applied to have her made a ward of court so that she could be sterilized. Leave was given by the court for the operation to proceed, but the Official Solicitor, representing Jeanette's interests, appealed. The case went before the Law Lords, who dismissed the appeal and the sterilization was allowed to proceed.

This was not a visual story. The family not having been identified meant that words took centre stage in the reporting of the case. The headline writers, as the report found, had 'a field day'. They came up with a wide variety of ways of devaluing the young woman, in particular, calling her 'Retarded Girl', 'Sex-risk girl', 'Tragic girl', 'Mental girl' and devaluing people with learning difficulties in general by calling them 'Retarded youth', 'Breed apart', 'Girls who mustn't be mums', and 'When childhood lasts a lifetime'. This case, involving sex, gender and disability revealed a whole viper's nest of prejudice: 'The sexuality of people with learning difficulties has always been a topic on which the Press and public alike have felt free to speculate or offer instant opinion'. Jeanette's story, the report found, 'provided just such a chance for journalists and letter-writers, many of whom were, it seemed, self-appointed experts. If the Press were to be believed, then "Everybody knows that Mentally deficient children are affectionate and outgoing, with the kind of warm, instinctive sexual responses of puppies"; and that "Some of the girls (with mental handicap) have strong sexual desires; and on the whole they are unable to control these needs"'.

Overall, the report found that Jeanette was portrayed as having, 'no redeeming features, no strengths, no preferences, no positive aspects to her personality'. It then adds the comment, 'If people with learning difficulties were ever to sue for character defamation there would surely be a case to pursue here'. Given the often inaccurate and conflicting comments in the Press, the report stated that, 'At times the newspaper reader must have found it hard to decide whether Jeanette was a teenage vamp looking for sexual adventures or a little girl who needed protection from the sexual advances of the rest of the world . . . despite the fact that she was neither of these'. Such attitudes towards women's sexuality have a very familiar ring to them.

The case of Jeanette was analysed separately from all the other press coverage of people with learning difficulties by Alison Wertheimer. She found that the term 'learning difficulties' had yet to reach the Press'. Not only had the Press not taken on board linguistic change, they revealed great ignorance and confusion about the difference between mental illness and mental handicap (learning difficulties). The report found that time and time again, journalists confused the two terms, sometimes using them as though they were interchangeable. The general findings were that people with learning difficulties get a 'poor press', depicted usually as objects of pity, often as eternal children, with the implication being that they are 'a race apart'. Newspaper reporters assumed that these people were 'poor souls who are unable to speak up for themselves', though, as this report points out, 'Nobody seemed to think of asking people with learning difficulties what they thought so they didn't get a chance to speak up'. Although, in general, the 'poor creatures' image dominated, the possibility that people with learning difficulties may be threatening and frightening also emerged, particularly in the coverage of a visit by the Princess of Wales to a centre for people with learning difficulties. There were many positive images in the coverage, but the Press could not refrain from commenting of the Princess that 'only once did she show any strain' . . . 'it could have been distressing' . . . and to the surprise of one journalist, 'the Princess appeared unperturbed'.

Terms this report did not mention, but ones that were used frequently in describing Down's Syndrome people were as 'high grade' or 'low grade'. They were terms I found deeply offensive. I quickly became aware that there is a wide range of abilities possessed by people who have an extra chromosome. Sometimes I would be told reassuringly, 'I am sure he will be high grade'. Far from being reassured, I felt that these well-meaning people were merely reinforcing their notion that Will belonged to a 'race apart' who, being barely human, could be graded. Another term, had I known about it then, I would have found equally offensive. A feature of Down's Syndrome, though not common to all – Will did not have it – is a single crease across the palms of their hands. As Brian Stratford explains in his book *Down's Syndrome Past, Present and Future*, 'This feature is known as the "simian" crease. "Simian" literally means pertaining to the apes or monkeys'. The term is a legacy from those in the medical profession who claimed 'mongolism' originated from a sub-animal species. 'However', as Brian Stratford points out, 'It is difficult to accommodate to this theory the fact that a fair percentage of the "normal" population also carry this distinctive crease!'

The use of language can be changed. The issuing of guidelines and the drawing up of linguistic codes of conduct can and do focus debate on the issue of language. Until people realize the need to change language; until they realize how obscene, offensive and discriminatory such language as, for instance, the language used in the coverage of the Jeanette case is then meaningful change will not happen. It is hardly surprising that of all the groups struggling for respect, those with learning difficulties have been the last to 'come out' and assert themselves. Those whose disabilities did not affect their ability to speak and articulate led the change and the others have followed. With all groups, be they women, gays, black people, people with disabilities, it has been each group of people themselves who have campaigned for change, not others on their behalf.

What is noticeable in the case of those with disabilities, particularly learning difficulties, is that parents have been central to the campaign. Parents who love, care and value their children and who have fought, and still fight, the rejection of their children by society have been integral to this change. Loving children with Down's Syndrome, as all the parents interviewed in Newham and others who speak or write about their experiences affirm, has made them fighters. One Newham mother described her change: 'I'm *never, ever* going to be frightened of anything again. Before I had Micky I would never say boo to a goose. But I think all the time where you have to keep on fighting all the time, so now, like you, get so mouthy in the end you can't shut up, you know (laughs), you end up winning the argument because you can't shut up, like. You've had to be like that all the time, otherwise you feel you ain't getting there, they're getting the better of you'. A father speaking of his personal transformation said, 'It has given me confidence. I'd never have gone out and do what I do now five years ago. I mean I find it hard, it's very hard now, because I haven't got the education, but it's a funny old world - I wouldn't have been a school governor or joined all those committees and spoken in public, things like that. I try to do things as best I can. I mean, now I will do these things: I have to. It's something you've got to do, if you can manage it. I think if we hadn't and other people hadn't, we wouldn't have got anywhere'.

THEORIES OF CHANGE

Experience, as so many testify, changes us as individuals and many become committed to bringing about wider change. My responses to the experience of Will were instinctive, fuelled by my immediate and deep love for him. The shock of finding such a contrast between what *I* felt about my son and what *society* felt about him has never left me. I wrote *Will, My Son* partly to express this deep shock; it was not in any way a theoretical book. I did not read any analysis of society's attitudes to those with learning difficulties or about how they could be changed. I knew how *I* wanted them changed. My experience as a woman who also wanted society's attitudes to myself and other women changed fed into my understanding. Having written *Will, My Son*, I retreated, as a survival mechanism, from involving myself directly in issues to do with those with learning difficulties.

When I started to research for this book, I knew the issues I wanted to follow up on - they were there in the original. Indeed, the brief I had given myself and the publisher was that issues raised in the original text of *Will, My Son* would be the starting off point for each section of this book.

In the seventies, opinions were changing. Segregation of those with learning difficulties was beginning to be questioned. Families were increasingly being encouraged to keep their child within the family and, thus, at some levels, within the community. After this first step other, changes have followed. They are no longer just ideas, they have been formalized within a legislative framework. Returning to the subject, I found that people had also developed new theories about society's attitudes to people with learning difficulties and these theories have informed, and continue to inform, how change should be achieved. The theories are to inform what and how steps should be taken to bring about acceptance of people with learning difficulties as part of our community.

When I visited Lucy Baxter, our time was largely taken up with me asking her a whole range of questions about herself, her decision to adopt two Down's Syndrome children and her experiences of other people's attitudes. Before leaving, she offered to lend me some material that she thought I might be interested in reading. She made little comment on it, except that it emerged that she was involved with the group Values Into Action and most of the material she lent me was published or distributed by them. There were things I knew would interest me. However, included was a booklet written by Wolf Wolfensberger entitled *A Brief Introduction to Social Role Volorization as a High-order Concept for Restructuring Human Services* and I politely accepted the loan of this booklet, privately thinking that it was the one piece of literature she had lent me that I would skip through.

Back at home, I decided that I should at least give this booklet a try. After all, it had been lent to me by Lucy, someone whose views, clearly, were close to mine, and she must have lent it to me for some reason. Somehow, one morning, I managed to get over my resistance to the language of the title and the equally impenetrable language used in the introduction, 'The Intended Purpose Of This Monograph'. Having read three pages, I was sure that this monograph was going to rival various film studies monographs that had been written when semiology was at the height of its intellectual vogue, so complicated were they, but, I thought, Lucy has lent this to me. I read on. To my surprise, I found that the main body of this monograph is in clear, concise, accessible language.

In it, Wolfensberger sets out a theoretical analysis of how societies value certain people and devalue others. As individuals, we have our own hierarchies of the people we value or devalue, but, as Wolfensberger points out, there is a 'second level of devaluation of people' that 'takes place on the level of a social collectivity and even an entire society, where entire classes of people are judged negatively by an entire collectivity, society or majority thereof'. It is this kind of devaluation that 'is most devastating, because it creates and maintains societally devalued classes who systematically receive poor treatment at the hands of their fellows in society and at the hands of societal structures - including formal, organized human services'. All these groups of 'others' - women, black people, gays and lesbians - will immediately recognize the truth of this observation. Others, too

- the poor, the unemployed, the old and the physically deformed - are devalued by a society that values youth, beauty and wealth. The creation of value systems is universal, but the particular elements of the value system are the product of each particular culture. A woman who could only hobble because she had grossly deformed feet would not be cast as a highly paid star in a Hollywood movie. Yet, for centuries in China, such grossly deformed feet, the product of foot binding, would have been seen as a sign of a woman's high class, value and beauty.

Wolfensberger, although explaining his theory in general terms, is concerned with how people are devalued because of disability. His aim is to bring about a change whereby, in particular, people with learning difficulties can become valued by society. This process of change he calls 'normalization' and explains it as, 'The utilization of culturally valued means in order to establish and/or maintain personal behaviours, experiences and characteristics that are culturally normative or valued'. My reaction to this statement was to ask the questions, should we not recognize difference and should we not change our cultural norms? Even if, I thought, it is a desirable aim, it is unachievable in practice. Yet, I know, from my experience of Will, that 'normalization' informed my actions. Like any mother of a newborn baby, I wanted him to look good and be well-dressed, but my feelings about how he looked went deeper. I remember buying what, in normal circumstances, I would have thought a ridiculously expensive outfit for a baby and thinking, 'If he is going to be accepted, he has to look good; people have to know I accept him, that I am proud of him'. When I received the literature from the Down's Babies Association, as it was called then, including physical and mental exercises drawn up by Rex Brinkworth, my response was one of relief.

Suddenly here was someone telling me of all the things I could do *for* my child and explaining *why* they needed doing and what the effect would be. Instead of reading lists of all the things which we should expect our child not to do and of all the physical and mental problems we could expect, here was someone saying 'we do not know what your child's potential is but it is almost certainly much greater than those about you have probably led you to expect'.

Underlying my relief was the feeling that I could take action that would develop Will's potentialities and, thus, make him more acceptable to and, thus, valued by society. Mentally, I went further in pursuing his normalization. The thought that he might be shunted away from society into a segregated school 'increased my resolve that I would do everything I could to help Will reach a level of development which would make him acceptable in a normal school'.

Given my own responses it is hardly surprising that, as I read through the areas Wolfensberger details as important in helping people with learning difficulties to be valued, I could only find myself agreeing with them. If someone is dressed in clean, well-fitting, appropriate clothes, it makes a huge difference to how they are perceived. Living accommodation – be it flats or a house – that is situated where other normal people live is to make a statement about the value of those living in that accommodation. Teaching people to eat in the most socially acceptable way they are capable of also makes sense. Recognizing someone's individuality and their desire to express their individuality is central to giving a person value. Changing the language we use to speak about and the images we use to portray people with learning difficulties are all part of the package of normalization.

My questions remained, however, even though I realized that Wolfensberger was expressing much of what I thought and felt. The intention of the theory is clear. Its aim is to empower people with learning disabilities and empowered people are valued.

A pamphlet designed for service workers, written by John O'Brien and Alan Tyne, called *The Principle of Normalization: A foundation for effective services*, directly confronts my, and clearly other people's, feelings, that the theory is based on the central contradiction that the principle of normalization says people with handicaps should be socially accepted and valued, but, isn't it devaluing handicapped people to try to make them normal? Although the theory *appears* contradictory, its actual practice is about bringing together. It is about bridging and lessening the gap between the valued and the devalued. For non-professionals, this means that each side is being brought closer to the other. Just as any attempt, however minimal, to speak the language of another country we visit is usually met with warmth and approval, attempts by people with learning disabilities to 'speak our language', either literally or in terms of behaviour, will elicit a positive or more positive response from us. It is in these interactions, these interrelationships, that better acceptance and understanding can grow. Each side of the relationship changes, lessening the divide and increasing understanding.

However, the theory of normalization is designed, largely, to inform the decision-making processes of service workers. It is designed to give those who provide services for people with learning difficulties a theoretical approach that, in practice, can be applied to a range of aspects of their work. It can inform anything from decisions about the design of living accommodation to the language of service workers and their ways of communication with their clients. It is stressed that normalization is '*not something that is done to a person. It is a principle for designing and delivering the services a person needs*'. As is explained, 'The principle of normalization is as practical as we are willing to work to make it. It sets a direction; it does not provide a highly detailed road map. It calls for increasing the probability that, over time, handicapped people will more and more live with us as valued neighbours than as devalued clients'.

The debate about the issue of whether or not difference should be made socially acceptable or rather, that every effort should be made to minimize it becomes at its most clear with regard to the question of cosmetic surgery. At birth, Will did not have the immediately recognizable features of a person with Down's Syndrome. The sister in the neonatal intensive care unit, although she had nursed and known several Down's Syndrome babies, told me that nothing in Will's features had caused her to suspect that he was Down's Syndrome. It was only as Will grew that the characteristic features began to be evident and then mainly when he was tired. Even then, *I* did not see *them*, I saw only my son. It was when looking at an image of him in a photograph, capturing him tired, with his face relaxed, that I saw the Down's Syndrome features. When fully awake and responsive, his face reflected his own personality, both in the flesh and in the image. The first time we had to really take on board the fact that Will would look different was when we met Tessa.

> The first impression was a shock. At the physical level Anna [Tessa] looked clearly Down's Syndrome with the immediately recognisable features and small stature. But like all abnormalities of looks, particularly not very marked ones and Anna's were not that marked, they soon recede on acquaintance as the individual's personality takes over.

The question of cosmetic surgery to make Down's Syndrome people look more normal was not one that I was aware of at the time of having Will though I now know that it was then already being pioneered.

There is a distinction between surgery that is primarily therapeutic and only secondarily cosmetic and surgery that is cosmetic in the sense of being designed to make someone look more 'normal'. Therapeutic surgery is that which would be considered for any child who has a defect that inhibits the functioning of part of their body and where the surgical intervention would improve that functioning. There is little division of opinion on the question of whether or not an operation to any child's nose that will make it easier for the child to breathe should be performed. However, the response to the idea of performing cosmetic surgery on a particular group of people to try to make them conform to some socially acceptable notion of normal looks would be quite different. In pursuing a course of plastic surgery, parents hope that, by making their child's looks conform more to notions of normality, their child will have a greater chance of being accepted by society.

When I started to read *Living In The Real World*, I was taken by surprise that the first chapter was on the subject of beauty. It made me realize that the issue of 'looks', one that had not existed in the mid-seventies when cosmetic surgery was not offered, is now a central one. The first statement in the book made by a parent is, 'I'm not considering cosmetic surgery for Marie, whatever. Because, you see, I think that if I can't accept Marie as she *is*, then the question must arise, why do I expect other people to accept her?' Reading on, it becomes clear that what is at issue regarding cosmetic surgery is this question of the acceptance of the child for who they are. All the parents interviewed in the book argue for the acceptance of difference. One mother puts forward the argument 'I mean I'm fat. I could lose weight. Why should I change? I can't see the point to it really. No one else changes, so why should Louise change? After all these years I don't see any difference, it doesn't affect me, in the way that they're people first and not Down's Syndrome, so I don't take any notice of what they look like. As I say, I've got a boy as well who's six foot two and a half and as skinny as a beanpole – you know, do I chop two inches off him to make him look a bit Mr Average?' Parent after parent, including myself, echoes the sentiment of one who said, 'Anyway, I love Leanne's face the way it is, and I wouldn't alter it'.

When I met Anya Souza, a young woman who has Down's Syndrome, one of the first issues that she raised was the question of cosmetic surgery. 'I like my face as it is', she said and added, 'There is nothing wrong with the way we look.' As Brian Stratford says in *Down's Syndrome Past Present and Future*, 'No reasonable argument can be put forward for changing the appearance of a child with Down's Syndrome in order that the child becomes more acceptable to the society in which he lives'. He goes on to add, 'If society finds it difficult to accommodate the child with Down's Syndrome, it is society which needs to change and not the child'. It is parents, however, who make decisions about whether or not a child should have cosmetic surgery. Over this the child has no control and the imposition, in the form of surgery, of notions of physical normality on a child should be questioned.

This said, adults should have the right to make decisions for themselves about what makes them feel and look better. Where does one draw the line and say that one form of cosmetic change is acceptable and another is not? It is a complicated area where our feelings about ourselves interface with the ever-changing social ideas about beauty. There are those who believe that we should go grey gracefully and accept what is natural, but there are others who determinedly defy nature, dyeing their hair. Women spend huge sums trying to remould their bodies to the currently held notions of slimness and beauty, while other women argue that difference should be accepted and that 'big is beautiful'. Men subject themselves to a range of treatments to try to stop themselves going bald or to replace lost hair. Our looks are important to most of us and, thus, are integral to our feelings of self-confidence. Although many of us question the excesses of people's attempts to conform to some image of beauty or to fight the process of ageing, most of us do care about our looks in terms of how we view ourselves and how we are seen by others. Most of us, though, perhaps not going so far as surgery, do make cosmetic alterations to ourselves in order that we may fit in with our ideas of culturally accepted views of physical appearance.

For people with Down's Syndrome to speak up and voice their own opinions on this issue, or, indeed, on any other issue, takes the whole debate into another realm. Until they started speaking for themselves, others – governments, charities, social services, the medical profession and parents – made decisions on the basis of what they, as experts, thought could and should be done for and to people with learning disabilities. The growth of self-advocacy is challenging all this. Self-advocacy – people with disabilities speaking for themselves about their needs and attitudes – is part of normalization. To find a voice in our society is to find a place within society. This voice has come as quite a shock to those who, often with the best of intentions, have dedicated their lives to caring for and helping those 'less fortunate than themselves'. In a television programme called *The Charity Business – People First*, broadcast in 1993, Matthew Griffiths, then Head of Education and Training at Mencap said, 'I think for many people, both parents and professionals, it came as quite a shock that people with learning difficulties had views. It is something we hadn't thought about and it is a challenge to one's thinking'. Other comments Matthew Griffiths made gave the impression that this was a challenge to which he could respond positively. However, it was clear that others in the charity business do not accept that the people they claim to represent have valid views of their own.

The group that has spearheaded self-advocacy in Britain is People First. Gary Boulet, influenced by the growing number of groups in the USA who were developing their own assertiveness skills, set up the first People First group in Britain in the mid 1980s. Since then, the movement has spread and groups have grown up across the country. In 1993, a decision was made to set up Young People First to help adolescents and young adults find their voice in the community. I had heard of People First when doing my research, but it was only when I went in to their head office to buy an information pack that I learned that one of the full-time organizers of Young People First was a woman, Anya Souza, who has Down's Syndrome. I knew that as part of my journey of discovery I had to meet her.

I phoned and, having explained what I was doing, asked if I could come in and meet her to find out more about her and her work. After I put the phone down, I was taken aback by the normality of the conversation. Between her engagements and mine, we finally settled on a mutually convenient time. The phone call was like any other 'normal' call making such an arrangement. My visit had the same normal air as had the phone call. We sat there together with her colleague and discussed the work of Young People First and the issues that are of particular concern to young people with learning difficulties. We discussed Anya's planned trip to Barcelona to speak to the Third International Conference on people with Down's Syndrome. Sitting there, talking with her about her life, living in her own flat left to her by her mother, and earning her living, one could not help but hold in one's mind what was said about her when she was born, that the doctor had told her mother in 1962, 'Your daughter will be physically and mentally handicapped for the rest of her life'.

Back home, I talked to my daughter, Jessie, about my experience. I told her of how, when we had Will, such a positive scene was unimaginable. I then went on to describe Anya, her life and work. Jessie then said to me, 'So why isn't she normal? I mean what's not normal about her'. I was left speechless for a moment by the obvious logic of her response. 'She *is* normal', I said, and added, 'She just has an extra chromosome'. 'So?', Jessie replied.

4 / To be or not to be

VALUE JUDGEMENTS

Attitudes to Down's Syndrome not only inform how people respond to the existence of this group of people who are genetically different, they also inform whether or not Down's Syndrome babies should be brought into existence and, once born, whether or not equal effort should be given to try to maintain their survival, as would be given to a normal child.

Prior to the invention of prenatal testing, there was no way of knowing whether or not a child would be born with Down's Syndrome until it was born. What was known then, however, is that the incidence rate is universal - class, race and culture have no influence. Hereditary factors also have no influence either, except in a tiny percentage of parents where Down's Syndrome has been caused by translocation. Maternal age is the one known influential factor, that the incidence increases with a mother's age. Most Down's Syndrome babies are born to mothers between 20 and 29, simply because most babies are born to mothers of that age. However, at the age of 25, the likelihood of having a baby with Down's Syndrome is 1 in 1500; by the age of 45, it is 1 in 30.

What is *not* known is how many babies born with Down's Syndrome were, and are, quietly left to depart this world without all known medical efforts being made to try to ensure their survival. Prior to the invention of antibiotics, respiratory infections were one of the main causes of death. Heart defects, in themselves or as a contributory factor to respiratory infections, were and are the other main cause of death. Greatly improved techniques of heart surgery have reduced the mortality rate attributed to this cause considerably. With the advances of medicine also came the dilemma as to whether or not they should be used to try to prolong a Down's Syndrome life. Medicine has developed the means to enable most to survive well into adult life, but the medical profession is not at all sure as to whether or not these means should be made available to people with Down's Syndrome.

This ethical issue is not one that I can muse over philosophically. I cannot stand back and argue that such questions are complicated ethical issues that require public debate. It is an issue that was presented to us starkly by a consultant cardiologist. Over the period of a few months, we had to take on board that Will not only had *a* heart defect, but a *serious* one. Following investigative surgery, we were told at the specialist heart hospital by the senior registrar, Dr Y, that, without surgery, Will's life expectancy would be brief. Surgery was, he stressed, high-risk, but, if successful, it would give Will a reasonable life expectancy. Without surgery, the prognosis was not good. By then, at seven months, Will's heart defect was affecting him physically. By this stage, his social development, in terms of laughing, smiling and responding to people around him, was advanced. He was also developing in other ways, gaining manual dexterity and hand–eye co-ordination, but:

> His physical development was quite definitely retarded. It was obvious he had a second handicap, a physical handicap, his heart. He was beginning to want to crawl and was trying to sit up but he had very little energy. He was quickly tired and became breathless from very little exertion. At that stage it was hard to work out what was due to physical handicap and what to mental handicap. Much less hard to work out was our reaction to this problem. Faced with his heart the problem about his mental handicap receded.

Surgery, Dr Y said, knowing us and Will, was what he would advise for a normal child, and this advice was couched in such a way that we knew it was what he advised for us. Before making our final choice, though, Dr Y felt we should discuss it with the consultant, Mr X. Of this discussion, I wrote:

> Dr Y explained briefly to him that he had told us what the situation was and that we would like to opt for the operation. Mr X then offered us a different perspective, one which shattered me. Up to this point we had been talking with Dr Y about our child

as any parents talks about a child that they love and cherish. There was an implicit assumption, shared by him, that parents want their child to live. Suddenly we were being offered a different option, of letting our child die. We found ourselves sitting there being told by Mr X that if we didn't want to choose the operation, that if, because of our child's handicap, we wanted them to leave our child (inevitably to die) they would respect our decision.

Fortunately, Dr Y quickly intervened, replying for us that he was sure the operation was what we wanted to choose and Mr X agreed that we should proceed with surgery.

We left the hospital shattered. We had just made a life or death choice for Will - one in which, in fact, we felt we had no choice. But much more shattering was the very stark way in which it had been brought home to us that our child was a second class human being in some people's eyes. It was most hurtful to realise that because he was a Down's Syndrome child leaving him to die was an option.

Transcribing this description evokes a sense of shock in me. The emotions are no longer so raw, but my sense of outrage has not mellowed.

Parents, in this situation, who do not, as we did, have absolute certainty in their attitude will be strongly influenced by the information given to them by doctors. Although the theory may be that doctors should, in these cases, provide parents with 'neutral' information the theory inevitably falls down in practice. For better or worse, doctors bring their own attitudes to such discussions, implicitly or explicitly. Shortly after Will died, I read an article in *The Guardian* about an interview with a consultant paediatric cardiologist, Dr Elliott Shinebourne. He talked about the great advances being made in Britain in children's heart surgery and went on to say that he did not 'personally believe that we should do all we can for a child that is maybe brain-damaged or mongol', and that he would not 'want to help keep a life if that child was going to be severely retarded'. Although Dr Shinebourne said that he responded to parents' wishes, he questioned 'whether with our fancy surgery we are keeping alive

babies whom nature would have let die?' Carol Dix, who had
conducted the interview, wrote sharply 'For most parents
involved the question is not so confusing. They know they want
to be able to defeat nature'. My comments on these statements
in *Will, My Son* were that I would have liked to have asked Dr
Shinebourne:

> What do you mean by nature? Is nature only to take its way with
> some children and not others? Is not the whole heart unit a superb
> example of our attempt to defeat nature? Mr Shinebourne, do you
> think you have the right to arbitrate on which part of nature
> should be defeated and which part should be left to take its way?

Until meeting Mr X, I had not realized that there were doctors
who believed that all efforts should *not* be made to try to ensure
the survival of my child. My GP had been very unsupportive
when I registered Will, so I had promptly changed to another
more sympathetic GP, but, otherwise, no other doctor - and I saw
many - gave any hint that they thought that any available
treatment on offer that might improve Will's condition would or
should not be offered him. With hindsight, I do not think this was
a case of me not 'hearing' what people were saying because I
didn't want to hear it. There is no one more sensitive to the
subtext of any comment than a parent when that comment is
about their child. From what I know now, I realize that we were
very lucky in our contacts with most medical professionals.
Although profoundly shocked by the attitude of Mr X, it was only
after Will's death that I realized that his attitude was, if not the
dominant attitude of members of the medical profession,
certainly one that was and is widely accepted.

One of the problems of trying to find out what attitudes people
have is that these decisions, like ours, take place in private
discussions. Mostly, the general public is never aware of the
decisions or, indeed, that these decisions are being made. In 1981,
however, the year *Will, My Son* was published, two highly
publicized cases *did* bring the subject out into the open, and
triggered extensive public discussion. Not surprisingly, I followed
them with strong feelings and deep emotions. When researching

for this book, I read Ann Shearer's *Everybody's Ethics: What future for handicapped.* Her booklet discusses the legal and ethical implications of both judgements. While reading it, the emotions that the cases triggered in me came back, vividly. The precise details, which I did not remember from the time, have been drawn from her booklet.

The first case was that of baby Alexandra. She was Down's Syndrome and, shortly after her birth, it was discovered that she had an intestinal blockage - quite a common complication of Down's Syndrome. An operation, if quickly performed, could have saved her life. Her parents refused to give their consent to it. The hospital referred the situation to their local authority, Fulham and Hammersmith, which made Alexandra a ward of court, gaining care and control, and gave authority for the operation to go ahead. Alexandra was moved to another hospital, but, there, the surgeon, hearing of the parent's wishes, refused to operate. Finally, the case went to the Appeal Court where Lord Justice Templeman ruled that it was wrong that a child's life should be terminated because, in addition to Down's Syndrome, she had another disability, and Lord Justice Dunn agreed, pointing out that there was no evidence that the child's life was likely to be an intolerable one. Alexandra had her operation and was, subsequently, fostered.

Later that same year, another case hit the headlines. The organization LIFE informed the police that a Dr Leonard Arthur had noted about a Down's Syndrome baby, John Pearson, in the presence of the babies parents, 'Parents do not wish it to survive. Nursing care only'. John Pearson died 69 hours after he was born of 'bronchopneumonia due to consequences of Down's Syndrome'. Dr Arthur was charged with murder; he denied the charge. At the trial, the defence claimed that the baby's physical complications were extensive and, therefore, it was not a simple case of Down's Syndrome. At the judge's direction, the charge was changed to that of attempted murder - a charge Dr Arthur was acquitted of by the jury.

In the course of this trial, it became clear, through evidence given in Dr Arthur's defence, that there was a degree of unanimity in the medical profession in support of Dr Arthur's decision. The view of Sir Douglas Black, President of the Royal College of Physicians, supported by others, was that 'It is ethical to put a rejected child with Down's Syndrome on a course of management that will result in its death; it is ethical that such a child suffering from Down's Syndrome should not survive'. After the trial, a leading article in the *British Medical Journal* stated, 'If the child is one of the quarter of newborns with Down's Syndrome with congenital defects of the heart or other internal organs, then treatment may reasonably be withheld if that is the consensus reached by the parents and at least two doctors'.

Confusion reigned in 1981 as a result of these two contradictory legal judgments. As Ann Shearer pointed out, 'Both children were rejected by their parents, but while their wishes were overridden in Alexandra's case in the best interests of the child, in this case [the case of John Pearson] parental rejection appeared, from the judge's direction to the jury, to become one of the criteria by which it was lawful to treat a baby with a sedating drug and offer no further care. His other criterion appeared to be that the child was "irreversibly disabled". Both Alexandra and John Pearson had Down's Syndrome. But Alexandra, who lived, was apparently *more* disabled than John Pearson, who died, for, at the time the decision not to treat was made, there seemed to be no indication that he was other than a normally healthy child'.

These two cases provoked extensive column inches in the newspapers and much television time was given to the issue. For a short period, attitudes were out in the open, revealing both deep divisions in society and also deep levels of ignorance and prejudice. Attitudes to Down's Syndrome were explicitly and implicitly clear in the debate. When all the flurry had died down, the central issues remained unresolved. Ian Kennedy, Director of the Centre of Law, Medicine and Ethics at King's College, was one who studied the implications of the Arthur case and, in summing up, he wrote in *New Society* (7 January, 1982), 'The ethical and legal implications which arise from the Arthur case are hard to face, let alone resolve, but we must do so. We owe it to our doctors, and to ourselves'.

In looking at the details of the cases, Ian Kennedy questioned making decisions on a diagnosis of 'irreversibly disabled', asking who should or can make such a certain prognosis. Doctors are influential in these situations, though their stated position at the time, expressed in the 1980 British Medical Association handbook of ethics, was that *'the parents must ultimately decide'.* However, society, as Ian Kennedy rightfully pointed out, cannot give parents the right to decide whether or not their child should live: 'It has never been part of our law or morality that parents may choose death for their children'. In 1983, the British Medical Association council approved an amendment to the handbook that underlines, instead, the rights of the *child*, asserting, 'A malformed infant has the same rights as a normal infant'. The trend since 1983 has been, increasingly, to put the rights of the *child* first. The current guidelines, *Medical Ethics Today*, issued by the British Medical Association, cite the case of Baby J in which the Appeal Court had recommended non-treatment on the grounds that 'the baby's existence would be painful and the benefits of the treatment continuing this painful existence would be minimal'. However, the handbook goes on to state, 'It was made clear in the *Re* J that the court's decision should not be seen as sanctioning widespread non-treatment of handi-capped neonates (or older children). The judges emphasised a generally strong presumption in favour of life and the need for substantial proof that the child faced a very poor quality of life before non-treatment could be considered. The criteria for quality-of-life judgements, it was said in *Re* J, should be what the child would choose "if he were in the position to make a sound judgement"'.

In practice, it would appear that these guidelines are not universally respected. The 'malformed infant', child or, indeed, adult does not have the same rights as a normal person when it comes to the question of medical treatment. Because decision making, except when it hits the headlines, is a private affair based on discussions between doctors and parents or patients it is hard to find out what is actually going on behind the closed doors of the consulting rooms. Small pieces of information surface occasionally, making one realize that, not only has little changed since 1975, but that, possibly, things have become worse. From the information available, what does emerge is that, when parents choose to try to prolong the life of their child, their decision is frequently not respected by doctors.

Paul Williams, in a speech given to the 1992 annual conference of the British Institute of Mental Handicap, recounted the case of one mother in search of heart surgery for her Down's Syndrome daughter, Maria. The mother, Celeste Hinds, was told by two consultant cardiologists that her daughter's heart condition was inoperable and that, 'Yes she would die prematurely'. Friends, however, told Celeste Hinds that they knew of someone who had taken their child, who had also been told in Britain that their child's heart condition was inoperable, to the Sick Children's Hospital in Toronto where the child's heart had been successfully operated on. Celeste Hinds phoned the Sick Children's Hospital in Toronto and was told by the doctor there, 'We operate on this defect here routinely each week', and added, 'There is no question of us not doing it; if we don't, these children die. It is major surgery but we have a 90 per cent success rate. The defect does occur in normal children as well as in children with Down's Syndrome, but in much smaller numbers. Of 100 consecutive operations we do to repair this defect, 80 will be on children with Down's Syndrome'. Celeste Hinds took the good news that her child had an *operable* heart defect back to her British cardiologist, whose response was, 'You don't want to be asking yourselves *where* it should be done, but *whether* it should be done at all'. She was then told that the operation *was* done at her local hospital, but, in the six years that her cardiologist had been there, it had only ever been done on normal children. His attitude was that the risks of the surgery were acceptable for normal children, who 'grow up to work, get married and have families'. When Celeste Hinds asked, 'But what about Maria and other children like her with Down's Syndrome?', her cardiologist just shrugged his shoulders. She went on to discover that, 'Of nine Paediatric Cardiology departments in Britain, only one is prepared to operate routinely on children with Down's Syndrome. As a result around 300 children with Down's Syndrome may be needlessly dying each year'.

Britain likes to take pride in itself as a developed nation. Last year, my nephew, Michael, spent three months in Malaysia as part of his medical training. On his return he told me that, resources being very limited in the hospital he worked in, a Down's Syndrome child would have no chance of having heart surgery. Michael was just old enough to remember his cousin Will and does so with affection. I wonder, however, how long it will be before he realizes that Britain is closer in practice to Malaysia than to Canada.

It was of interest to me, too, to learn what other medical students thought about this issue. Dr Jane Bernal read to the class of students at St George's both the description of the choice we were given as to whether or not we wished to proceed with surgery and our reactions to being offered such a choice. Dr Bernal then asked the students whether or not they felt such decisions would still be presented in the same way. It was a question the students found difficult.

It was agreed in the discussion that it was proper to involve the parents in the decision and they felt that a consultant should not 'make an assumption about what the parents think and feel', but, rather, should make an attempt to find out where 'the parents are coming from'. Of the central issue, one student said, referring to our consultant cardiologist, Mr X, 'I think it was fair of him to make that point. Obviously the way in which he made it was important and how he came across to the parents but it was fair. You have to put all the options, all the points of the argument to somebody'. There was general agreement to this point. I found it quite shocking that not *one* student raised the question of whether or not leaving a Down's Syndrome child to die was an acceptable option. For me, and for many others, the inclusion of such an option as 'fair' raises profound ethical questions.

The debate about ethics, however, has, increasingly, been taken over, or, rather, represented, as a result of questions about cash since the creation of the internal market in the National Health Service.

Dr Bernal made this connection by raising the question, 'What determines the quality of somebody's life?' – a question that is now an integral part of the decision-making process of the National Health Service, as Celeste Hinds had found out when trying to ensure surgery for her child's heart. 'Quality-adjusted life years' are now the basis for decisions. Whether or not a procedure is funded is not just a matter of what it costs but what it delivers in terms of 'quality-adjusted life years'. Given a finite budget for health care, these difficult decisions are inevitable.

> If we are to accept the reality that decisions must be made as to what society can provide, or rather wishes to provide, in terms of health care, then the question is who should make those decisions?

The only change that has occurred since I wrote these words in *Will, My Son* has been that more decisions are made as to who gets what health care. Rationing of health care goes on increasingly, every day, in every sector of the Health Service. The question now, as then, is how these decisions are made and, most crucially, who makes them? The students could not think their way out of their own world of decision making, that is, as something concerning the individual doctor and patient rather than something society in general should concern itself with. They evaded this wider area of discussion, despite Dr Bernal raising a number of questions about it. The practice of medicine for them, informed, I am sure, by training in the enclosed world of a hospital, was about *the* doctor and *the* patient. When they do qualify, they will quickly realize, I have no doubt, that the reality of the practice of medicine is circumscribed by economic decisions.

These economic decisions are based on assessments of 'quality-adjusted life years'. How many 'quality-adjusted life years', one wonders, will a Down's Syndrome person be awarded and who will award such a rating? Clearly, in our case, we would have given one rating to the value and quality of Will's life, while our consultant cardiologist would have given another. Among our relatives, friends and acquaintances we quickly sensed what value rating they would give him just as we quickly sensed the different value ratings the various health professionals we met would give. What we learned, however, was that those who had become close to Will, who had held him, who had played with him, who had been warmed by his laughter had, like us, undergone change. Will, for them, like us, had become not a category of the human species – Down's Syndrome – but a person who was valued. In deciding on whether or not a chance for a future for Will (or the Will's of today) should be given, who should make this choice and on what information are they making such a choice?

Such decisions should involve *all* of us, just as decisions about who gets a kidney transplant should be made by society. They should not be made behind closed doors in private discussions; they should not be left to doctors or parents or economists. Difficult as they are, they are decisions that concern us all. In 1983, a number of major American organizations representing disability *and* medical interests together produced a statement, *Principles of Treatment of Disabled Infants*. At its core is the basic principle, clearly stated, that 'Discrimination of any type against any individual with a disability/disabilities, regardless of the nature or severity of the disability, is morally and legally indefensible'. It asserts that disabled people should have equal rights of citizenship, including health care, and that these rights should be recognized from birth. Translating this idea into actual practical guidelines means that whenever medical care is clearly beneficial, 'A person's disability must not be the basis for a decision to withhold treatment', and, 'When doubt exists at any time whether to treat, a presumption always should be in favour of treatment'. However, they state quite categorically that, 'It is ethically and legally justified to withhold medical and surgical procedures which are clearly futile and will only prolong the act of dying'. These guidelines form a good basis on which to discuss and develop a similar set of principles that should be respected in the UK.

The Patient's Charter, issued by the British Government in 1991, states very clearly that, 'Every citizen already has the following National Health Service rights'. The first of these existing rights is 'To receive health care on the basis of clinical need, regardless of ability to pay'. Clinical need of *every* citizen, therefore, is the basis for treatment. The Charter goes further and states that, 'There are nine standards of service which the

NHS will be aiming to provide for you'. The first two of these standards are 'Respect for privacy, dignity and religious and cultural beliefs' and 'Arrangements to ensure everyone, including people with special needs, can use the services'. There is nothing in the Charter that says, if you have an extra chromosome, you are not a citizen and, therefore, do not have equal rights to be treated on the basis of clinical need. Besides the cases of young children being refused heart surgery, the Down's Syndrome Association know of recent cases of young adults having been turned down for major surgery on the grounds that they have Down's Syndrome. In these cases, we are not dealing with what, for most, are difficult ethical issues about whether or not a newborn baby may have a life of severe disability and suffering ahead of it, we are dealing with people who are living their lives and who could live their lives more productively and with less suffering if they were given the treatment they need, treatment that would not be refused them if they had 46 chromosomes.

THE NEW FRONT LINE

The debate in 1981, triggered by the two cases involving giving treatment to or withholding it from Down's Syndrome babies, at least brought these issues out into the open. It is hard to know whether or not the debate has died down simply because no new cases have brought the issue into the public spotlight or because attitudes have changed. What has definitely changed over the past 20 years, though, is that the front line of these ethical issues has moved. It has moved forward to the testing of foetuses for abnormalities. In this move forward in the cycle of human life, society appears to have moved even further backwards in its refusal to take responsibility for tackling the ethical issues that this advance in medical technology has given rise to.

The first time I heard of testing the foetus for chromosomal abnormalities was shortly after Will had been diagnosed as Down's Syndrome. My obstetrician told me that if I became pregnant again, he would offer to perform an amniocentesis so that the possibility of Down's Syndrome could be averted in a second pregnancy. At the time, a day or two after Will's diagnosis, it seemed a reassuring piece of information. When I did become pregnant again, about a year after Will's death, the knowledge that I could be tested for a chromosomal abnormality was no longer simply reassuring; I had been changed by love for my son. Making the decision whether or not to be tested was difficult for me.

> The amniocentesis was offered me on the assumption that if anything were found to be abnormal I would agree to a termination of my pregnancy. In fact it was spelt out to me that they perform the test on the understanding that a termination would be carried out if anything was wrong.

I was told that the test carried with it the risk of provoking a miscarriage. This was a risk I considered seriously as I desperately wanted another child. This consideration the medical profession understood and they tried hard to reassure me that the risk was small. My other concerns were, I felt, so far from their (and most other people's) capacity to understand I never even expressed them until writing *Will, My Son*. For me, in considering whether or not to have an amniocentesis:

> There was another much more difficult problem for me related to the test, a psychological one. If everything was found to be all right then it would be easy but if anything was wrong and in particular if the foetus present a Down's Syndrome chromosome structure what would I do? It was a problem few understood. Like the obstetricians, most people assumed that I would want to terminate the pregnancy. It was an assumption founded on their attitudes towards me and the handicapped; attitudes which varied from, at one extreme, those who assumed sympathetically that I would not want another handicapped child because of all the problems it would cause, and those, at the other extreme, who believe we should use the development of medical science to ensure the reproduction only of 'normal' people. From people's assumptions I realised they would regard it as irresponsible of me to knowingly bring another handicapped child into the world. If I did it would have been my decision and would then have to be my responsibility. I should not expect others to offer the support and help which they had offered to us and Will. On the other hand

> I knew that if I made the decision to terminate the pregnancy of a Down's Syndrome foetus I would be betraying Will. I would feel as though I was betraying not only him but all that I had fought for, for him and by implication for others like him - his right to a chance of life, to an education, to a place in society, to human dignity.

I did have the amniocentesis. It revealed no chromosomal abnormality. There is still a part of me that feels that the act of choosing to have an amniocentesis was an act of betrayal. My private personal ethical dilemma was one that should have been addressed by society. In returning to the subject, I wondered how much concern was now expressed about the issues. I found that, among certain sections of people, those with Down's Syndrome, those who are involved in their care and some geneticists, there is deep concern about prenatal testing. Pregnant women are also increasingly voicing their concerns. The number of women tested has increased greatly since 1977, when I was tested, as have the number of people concerned. There is little evidence, however, that there are many people who think what is going on is an ethical issue of sufficient importance to give it a public airing.

To me it appeared deeply ironical that, at the very time attitudes to Down's Syndrome people were changing and the campaign for their rights to equal citizenship was getting off the ground, modern medical science developed a technique for testing foetuses enabling decisions to be made as to whether or not Down's Syndrome people should be brought into existence. This double-think of society is succinctly summed up by Theresa Marteau in *Antenatal Diagnosis of Fetal Abnormalities* (Edited by J. O. Drife and D. Donnai, Springer-Verlag, 1991) in which she states, 'At the same time as encouraging a more positive environment for people with severe handicaps, resources are spent on preventing their births'.

There are two interrelated issues surrounding prenatal testing. One is the actual practice of it, what is going on in antenatal clinics. The other is the wider issue informing that practice, the issue of attitudes to people with learning difficulties.

To date, foetal testing can detect less than 50 per cent of birth abnormalities. These tests are able to detect, with differing levels of reliability, a number of chromosomal and genetic disorders. These include the more commonly known disorders, such as spina bifida and anencephaly, along with lesser-known diseases, such as Tay-Sachs Disease and Hurler Disease. However, Down's Syndrome forms the largest group of abnormality that can be diagnosed by prenatal testing. Unless a pregnant woman has a known family history of a particular hereditary condition for which there is a prenatal test, Down's Syndrome is what women are being offered a test to diagnose. It is because it forms the largest group of diagnosable foetal abnormalities, because testing for Down's Syndrome is what obstetricians offer pregnant women and because attitudes are divided about 'the value' of a Down's Syndrome life so that attention is focused both in antenatal clinics and by others on this area of prenatal testing.

At the moment, the only certain way of testing for the presence of Down's Syndrome in an unborn child is by taking a sample of foetal cells, then growing them in a laboratory until they are large enough for the chromosomes to be identified. Amniocentesis, which involves inserting a fine needle into the womb and removing some of the amniotic fluid which contains cells from the baby, is the only accurate test. No test guarantees a 100 per cent accuracy, but amniocentesis comes close. Carrying out the test, however, brings with it a risk of miscarriage and cannot be done much before the sixteenth week of pregnancy. It can then take up to four weeks before the results are available. Chorionic villus sampling, which removes a piece of the placenta using a fine tube inserted into the neck of the womb, gives about a 95 per cent accurate result. The advantage of this latter test is that it can be done much earlier in the pregnancy (about the eighth or tenth week), though it brings with it a higher risk of miscarriage than does amniocentesis.

Because of the risks involved in carrying out both these tests, they are usually only offered to mothers who, because of their age (usually 35 years plus), are more likely to have a baby with Down's Syndrome. Medical science has continued, and continues, to search for safer tests that can be done earlier on in a pregnancy.

The latest developments involve tests of the mother's blood. The results from these tests, which measure a number of different substances in the mother's blood, can only indicate whether or not a mother has a 'risk likelihood'. This 'risk likelihood' is measured in terms of in the range of a figure of 1 in up to 250 or above: 1 in a figure under 250, the risk is rated as low; 1 in a figure above it, is seen as high. If the tests reveal that the mother comes into the category of high risk, she will be offered either an amniocentesis or chronionic villus sampling. An even more recent development in early testing is the use of high-definition ultrasound scanning.

Theoretically, testing should be offered in a way that enables the parent(s) to make an informed choice. This requires that the mother (and father, if involved) has all the necessary information about any test. It also requires that the options following a positive result to a test are given to them in a manner that does not coerce them into making a particular choice. In my case, I was given the information I needed about the test by the obstetrician – what the procedure involved and that there was a risk of miscarriage. However, the offering of an amniocentesis on the basis that a termination would be expected if the results revealed any abnormality could hardly have been seen as allowing the patient, me, to give informed consent. Indeed, consent was required before I had the information.

Since 1977, when I was tested, prenatal testing has become much more widespread. Amniocentesis – something almost none of my friends had heard of when I had the test – is now available in all the 15 health regions of England and Wales. How routinely it is carried out is not known. Recent research, however, has revealed the ways obstetricians in one London teaching hospital present amniocentesis to women eligible because of their age. The results of this research, conducted by the Health Psychology Unit of the Royal Free Hospital, were published in 1993 in the *Journal of Reproductive and Infant Psychology* and they make fascinating reading.

The survey was based on tape-recorded consultations. The participants, having agreed to have the consultation tape-recorded, the researcher would turn the tape recorder on and leave the room. Because this method of research was used, the results not only provide statistical information of the presentations but also actual dialogue, vividly capturing the language used in such consultations.

In general, they found that their research highlighted 'The lack of training for obstetricians in presenting complex information about prenatal testing in ways compatible with informed consent'. To put it more bluntly, they found that, all too often, obstetricians gave the pregnant women little information, misinformation and presented the options in a non-neutral way. Informing the obstetricians' approach to women, the survey found that 'Implicit in obstetricians' presentations was a positive attitude towards the use of amniocentesis in routine pregnancies in older women. An assumption that all women would or should undergo the procedure was also evident'.

From 'listening in', they found that obstetricians' attitudes to amniocentesis often informed the language and the statistics they used. The report states that, 'All doctors described probabilities as risks. The probability of miscarriage tended to be described as low; while similar probabilities of having an abnormal baby tended to be described as high. A miscarriage rate of 1 in 100 was variously described as small, very small, and very rare. By contrast, risks of 1 in 120 and 1 in 160 for a baby with Down's Syndrome were described as high'. No doctor in this survey described what Down's Syndrome was, nor any of the other foetal abnormalities (mentioned only to some expectant mothers) that could be detected by the test. Down's Syndrome accounts for only about 50 per cent of foetal abnormalities that can be diagnosed by amniocentesis. The following is one doctor's comment – high on reassurance, low on information – in offering an amniocentesis: '. . . it doesn't guarantee you a normal baby but it does exclude some of the more common abnormalities which are associated with us ladies as we get a bit older and we have our babies'.

Given the attitudes revealed in the presentation of 'risks', it is hardly surprising to find that, although some doctors offered the test accepting that a woman could make a decision based on the result, others made it explicit that termination, if foetal abnormality were found, was one of the terms under which amniocentesis would be conducted. The divide between allowing women the right to choose based on the information acquired from the test and those who feel that this right should not be available stems from a difference of opinion on why prenatal testing is conducted in the first place. The authors of this survey lay out the two positions, stating, 'There is disagreement as to the purpose of presenting prenatal screening tests. While some hold with the view that the purpose is to reduce birth abnormalities (Wald, 1991), others have argued that the purpose of presenting prenatal screening is to provide prospective parents with information about the tests to facilitate an informed decision about their use (Royal College of Physicians, 1989)'. Putting the argument in cash terms, there are those who believe that resources should not be wasted on the whims of women who want to exercise the right to informed consent. The health visitor who wrote a hostile reader's report on *Will, My Son* said of my ambivalence about having an amniocentesis, 'I think most medical and nursing staff would have found the author's arguments about amniocentesis quite illogical. It ill behoves her to complain of lack of resources when she might have been prepared to waste them'. From recent evidence, it would appear that many health visitors, obstetricians and nursing staff today share her attitude.

There are a few women who, for a number of reasons or beliefs, are sure that they do *not* want to be tested. Only 2 women of the 25 women surveyed by the team from the Royal Free Hospital's Health Psychology Unit refused an amniocentesis. The obstetricians' responses in both cases reveal how difficult it is for women who do not have absolute confidence in their own choice of action to pursue their own wishes. In one case, 'Seemingly, in an attempt to dissuade a 40-year-old woman from declining amniocentesis, the doctor presented the probability of Down's Syndrome as twice as high as it actually was'. In the other case, the doctor, having presented the risk of having a Down's Syndrome baby as higher than the risk of having a miscarriage asked, 'What would you feel if you had a baby with Down's syndrome?' To which the woman replied 'Well, I'm a Nursery

Nurse. I have worked with all types of children so therefore it wouldn't be the end of the world'.

The evidence from other sources confirms that it is hard to say 'no' to being tested. Caroline Hearst wrote in *Everywoman* (June, 1990) of her experience of saying 'no'. She became pregnant at 35 and, because of her age, was offered an amniocentesis, which she refused. She also refused an alpha-fetoprotein test, which is a test of the mother's blood to see if there is a high probability that the foetus has spina bifida or anencephaly. 'I had to explain', she wrote, 'That I didn't really want a termination, regardless of the result of the test. I was terribly apologetic because I didn't want to get a reputation as a "difficult patient"'. Caroline Hearst did not want a late termination and that overrode her knowledge that 'Life with and for a mentally handicapped child can be isolated and grim'. Of the situation in general, Caroline Hearst wrote, 'In hospitals and doctors' surgeries up and down the land, pregnant women are being offered tests which presuppose our willingness to have abortions - and late ones at that, at 20 weeks or more. I found well-meaning medical personnel assuming that I would want these tests, and I experienced their incredulity, when I declined, as pressure to conform to their expectations'. In saying 'no', Caroline Hearst was aware that, given the pressure from her partner and from the medical profession, had she given birth to a child with a disability, it would be regarded as a 'wilful decision' on her part and one for which she could not expect support.

Prior to the development of a blood test that indicates 'risk likelihood', prenatal testing was confined to a small group of pregnant women - either those who, because of hereditary factors, know they are at high risk of having a baby with a severe abnormality or those, who because of maternal age, are more likely to have a baby with Down's Syndrome. New tests are changing all that. 'New method of screening cuts Down's baby risk', announced the *Independent* on 14 August, 1992. According to the article, the doctors from St Bartholomew's Hospital, who developed the test, thought 'All pregnant women should be offered the test, regardless of their age'. These same doctors viewed this new screening method as 'practical, acceptable and cost-effective'. In case anyone questioned their latter assertion, the researchers had costed their screening method and estimated that 'It costs £38000 to avoid one Down's baby. The lifetime cost of caring for one Down's child have been estimated at £120000'. The researchers are clearly unaware that some Down's Syndrome people are employed and, therefore, taxpayers. Indeed, the American TV star Chris Burke almost certainly pays more taxes than a medical researcher at St Bartholomew's Hospital. Just in case anyone, like me, might be profoundly shocked by the researchers' reduction of the value of a life to a sum of money, the doctors reassured us all that, 'The most important reason for screening, however, is not financial: it is the avoidance of handicap and of distress to the families concerned'.

The even more recent form of diagnosing Down's Syndrome, by ultrasound scanning, is currently being developed by Dr Kypros Nicolaides at King's College Hospital. He hopes that, by the end of the year, 20 000 women will have been scanned in order to confirm his results. Like the researchers from St Bartholomew's, Dr Nicolaides claims that the current practice of restricting screening to older women is missing the large numbers of Down's children born to younger mothers.

These recent developments mean that many more women now experience some form of testing. These tests often leave women confused, anxious and pressured. Too often, women lack the information on which to make a decision – indeed, sometimes they are not even informed that they are being tested for certain 'risks'. Currently, the Down's Syndrome Association receives more phone calls relating to prenatal screening than for any other reason. Most of the phone calls they receive are from pregnant women who have had a blood test or one of the high definition scans and have found that they are in the high-risk group. Under pressure to have an amniocentecis, with a termination as the assumed outcome if any abnormality is found, the women are looking for advice and counselling. They are in a state of anxiety, stress and indecision. Most simply want information that is as neutral as possible, so that they can make an informed decision for themselves. My experience of my friends and of monitoring their pregnancies is that a few are absolutely certain of their position. There are those who are sure they do *not* want a test and will 'take what comes', and those who want to be tested for every eventuality and, with equal certainty, would terminate the pregnancy if there was any evidence of abnormality, but they are in the minority. Most occupy a middle ground of uncertainty, conflicting feelings and emotions and wish that at such a time of emotional vulnerability, they were not put into the front line of ethical decision making.

The results of the tests, like the way they are presented, too often also come with a similar lack of explanation and information. Thus, a negative result can be interpreted by the prospective mother, if she is not properly informed, as a belief that everything is all right. Further, not only do these tests *not* detect over 50 per cent of birth abnormalities, the early blood tests are, in themselves, only indicators. The cut-off point of 250 is itself imprecise, too. Pat Evans described in *The Guardian* how her blood test revealed that her 'risk likelihood' was 1 in 260 and so was offered no further tests. Though not totally confident that everything was all right, she was only slightly worried. After her baby son was born, he was diagnosed as having Down's Syndrome.

There are further problems. Even when a definite diagnosis of a foetus is made, for many conditions, there is no way in which the doctors can predict how mildly or severely affected the child may be. In some cases, the known prognosis is that the child will suffer from severe abnormalities and will not survive beyond early infancy. However, being able to make a prognosis with such certainty applies to the minority of children born with genetic and chromosomal abnormalities. For most, the prognosis is much more open to probabilities and possibilities. The history of children with disabilities who have achieved a whole range of skills and abilities is the history of parents who have refused to accept and believe the negative prognosis given by doctors at the birth of their child. At present, although doctors can diagnose Down's Syndrome, they can only tell that the baby has an extra chromosome; they cannot, at that stage, diagnose whether or not there are other physical complications, such as a congenital heart defect. As for the baby's potentialities, there is no way of knowing what they might be. Under the umbrella term 'Down's Syndrome people' there is a wide range of abilities and personalities, just as an enormous range exists for normal people. The least predictable thing is how the parents will respond to the existence of their child in the fullness of time. The 'distress' caused by finding out the diagnosis is a distress witnessed by the doctors at the time of the telling, but what is clearly *not* witnessed by the doctors is the profound love that many parents have for their child within a very short time of its arrival into the world. Although a few Down's Syndrome children are put up for adoption (as, indeed, are normal children), the majority are loved and cherished by their families. In fact, there is a waiting list of parents who would like to adopt Down's Syndrome babies. Whether this is because more are now kept by their parents or fewer are born it is hard to know.

Those concerned about the practice of prenatal testing – what is actually going on in hospital consulting rooms – argue that ways need to be developed to ensure that information and counselling are given to pregnant women in a 'non-directional' manner – 'non-directional' being the giving of information, options and counselling in a non-evaluative and non-judgemental way. The aim is to ensure that pregnant women and their partners can make an informed choice, free from coercion, both as to whether or not they wish to be tested and, then, if they do opt to be tested, what action they wish to take following the findings. Research reveals that, in most hospitals, the practice falls far short of this aim. Indeed, it appears that many health professionals do not even share this aim. The Royal College of Obstetricians and Gynaecologists, for example, have not issued any guidelines to their members as to how any prenatal screening programmes should be conducted.

Mr John Friend, a practising obstetrician and spokesperson for the College, presents quite a different view to that revealed by research of how the practice of prenatal screening should be carried out. He stressed that women should 'opt in' and not have to 'opt out' of any prenatal screening programme. A woman, he said, 'Should be given the information relevant to her situation to entitle her to make her decisions'. Of the question of amniocentesis being offered on the basis of agreeing to a termination if any foetal abnormality was revealed, he said quite categorically, 'No way can we deny women the option to refuse termination'. The offering of amiocentesis routinely to women over 35 he questioned, on the basis that, by doing so, because of the miscarriage rate, a percentage of normal babies are miscarried. His 'hopes', however, lie in the development of an early blood test, currently being researched, that can isolate foetal cells in the mother's blood. This he sees as the safe, non-invasive way forward for prenatal testing.

The principles that should inform the practice of prenatal testing expressed by Mr John Friend would go some way towards ensuring women are able to give informed consent to any prenatal test if they were enshrined in a set of guidelines issued by the Royal College of Obstetricians. The underlying problem, however, is in the explicit and implicit attitudes of most obstetricians. In their enthusiasm for prenatal testing, it is clear that a high percentage believe they are doing a service to society in preventing the births of people with Down's Syndrome.

The issues relating to prenatal testing can no longer be dismissed as being issues concerning the few – if they ever could. As Theresa Marteau points out, 'The availability of prenatal screening and diagnostic testing has changed the experience of pregnancy. Before the development of prenatal testing for fetal abnormality, the fetus was assumed to be healthy, unless there was evidence to the contrary. The presence of prenatal testing and monitoring shifts the balance toward having to prove the health or normality of the fetus'. This pressure 'to prove the health or normality of the foetus' has implications far beyond decisions made privately in the hospital consulting room.

As a society, we are currently upholding two contradictory moral positions in relation to Down's Syndrome. On the one hand, we now, through changes in the law, are increasingly encouraging the integration of Down's Syndrome children into mainstream schooling. We support in principle (though often not in practice) their rights to employment and rights as citizens. At the same time, in effect, we support the prevention of their births. This contradiction is nowhere more glaring than in the June 1993 issue of *Mencap News*. Most of the magazine is devoted to articles that report positively about people with learning difficulties. In it, you can read about 'Integration in Germany – The Way Forward', of the inclusion in the AMICI dance theatre company of a performer with severe physical deformities and of a group of prisoners that 'has set up a unique project, to provide canal activity holidays for children with disabilities and chronic illnesses'. In it there is also a double-page spread entitled 'Watching Westminster' in which one can read reports of the lobbying activities of Mencap in relation to various pieces of relevant legislation, including a report headed, 'Petitions Support Civil Rights (Disabled Persons) Bill'. With no obvious consciousness of any contradiction, on page 3 there is an article headed, 'Early Scans Advised for the Detection of Down's Syndrome'. It reports another advance in the search for a method of safe, accurate and early detection of foetuses with Down's Syndrome. If I was a literate Down's Syndrome member of Mencap, I wonder what I would think and feel if I read that article, printed by an organization that claimed to represent my interests. Talking to Steve Billington, Mencap's Director of Marketing and Appeals, I asked him if Mencap had developed any guidelines or, indeed, had debated the ethical issues relating to prenatal screening. He responded that they had not and that when he was asked about the issue, he was 'quiet and pragmatic'. The Down's Syndrome Association, in contrast, expresses quite clearly their position: 'The Down's Syndrome Association and the parents it represents do not believe that having a baby with the condition is a reason to terminate a pregnancy. However, we realize that this is a decision for individuals to make'.

In all this debate, one voice is *not* heard; one opinion is *not* solicited – the opinion of those people with Down's Syndrome. It is not easy to sit there and ask someone with Down's Syndrome whether or not they think people like them should not be born, but I found myself in this position. It was a question I didn't want to ask. It was, I thought, an obscene question to ask, but I felt it should be asked if only to give people with Down's Syndrome a chance to speak for themselves.

The person I asked was a young woman I mentioned earlier – Anya Souza, who works for the group Young People First. As a

Down's Syndrome person, Anya has experienced the cruelty of people in the street calling her names and has been aware that many have viewed her as someone with very limited abilities. She has a resilient attitude to such slights, but I could feel her distress as I asked for her views on this issue. Before I left, she gave me a copy of a letter in which she was replying to a doctor who had asked for her views on prenatal testing. Anya's thoughts on the subject are simple and clear. She wrote, 'If people have an abortion they are saying the baby is worthless and will never be able to do anything, but just look at me now - I'm bright, I've got a good sense of humour, I have a full-time job and I socialise'.

Outside of those directly concerned, this is an issue about which society remains curiously quiet. There was a brief flurry of media attention triggered by the announcement in 1993 that scientists in the USA had discovered 'a linkage between a small region of one chromosome and sexual orientation in men'. This 'small region of one chromosome' got dubbed by the Press as the 'homosexual gene' and, over a short period of time, a large number of column inches were devoted to the question of prenatal genetic screening. Most focused on whether or not homosexuality was a case of nature or nurture and if the former, even in part, then the arguments of the moral majority could be silenced. Nature, presumably in the form of God, not sin, was the progenitor of homosexuality. Most journalists left the subject, reassured that this form of genetic screening was not only a long way off, but, also, was unlikely to ever be used as it could only reveal 'a linkage'.

Few journalists, however, used this story to widen the issue, to make any serious comment about prenatal screening - what is already practiced and what may become practice in the imminent future.

An editorial in *The Independent On Sunday* (18 July, 1993) was one of the few that did. In a leader entitled 'The genetic tyranny', the leader writer pointed out that, 'This is not an issue for homosexuals alone. One in 30 children is born with a genetic problem of some kind - blindness, deafness, mental handicap, for example. Perhaps we can accept the rights of their parents to decide that these are handicaps with which they would rather not cope. But what of the gene that predisposes to cancer or heart disease? Can we tolerate the idea that a parent might abort a child because it has a 50 per cent chance of dying at 45? If not, would we find it more tolerable if the chances were 95 per cent'. The article points out that, as research into the genetic component of many conditions speeds ahead gathering more and more information the question is, 'Where and how to draw the line?' The article ends with a warning that, 'tthe age of the 'designer baby' is probably less than two decades away' and suggests that 'Precisely because the problems are so dauntingly complex, some kind of public debate is urgent'.

We should learn from the experience of another country. In India, many girl babies are killed at birth. Although the practice is illegal and, in the eyes of the law, is murder, it is quite widespread. However, because social attitudes support this form of murder, few law enforcement agencies even try to prosecute offenders. With the development of ultrasound scanning, the sex of the foetus can now often be detected in pregnancy and the ultrasound scanning business is booming in India. It is estimated that 3000 girl foetuses are aborted every day in India following a sex determination scan. Most people in Britain who watched the BBC Assignment programme *Let Her Die*, I am sure, were shocked by the use of murder of a live infant or the termination of a pregnancy as a way of limiting the population of females. Like many others, I was shocked, but I was also struck by the similarity of arguments used by those who justify control of the population of girls to those who justify control of the population of people with Down's Syndrome. First and foremost was the economic argument. Girls are seen by parents as a high-cost bad investment. Money is seen as wasted on bringing them up only then to have to pay huge sums of money in a dowry payment, the new husband and his family reaping the benefits of their investment. One clinic advertising ultrasound scanning for sex determination stated on its billboard, 'Pay 500 rupees now. Save 50 000 rupees later'. It is the same economic logic of the St Bartholomew's research team. However, poverty and the cost of a girl child is not the heart of the matter. Rich families also value sons and see little value in daughters, and, indeed, rich women were the first to go to the ultrasound scanning clinics for sex determination tests.

One doctor, defending his practice of ultrasound scanning, explained that Indian people viewed the birth of the first girl as bad luck, the second as a disaster and the third as a catastrophe. In his clinic, we saw him scanning a woman and, having got the image on his screen, he says to her 'It is only a girl'. The mother responded by revealing, through her tears, that this was bad news and, because she, her family and society did not want or value girls, the pregnancy would be terminated. A response similar to that of many women on being told that their foetus has 47 chromosomes.

In *Let Her Die*, there were two sequences shot in a maternity hospital that poignantly highlighted the difference in the value attached to the birth of a boy and of a girl. One scene was of a mother who had just given birth to a son by caesarean section - the surgery was not clinically needed, but had been performed just to ensure *his* absolute safe delivery. She was surrounded by her whole family. They were all smiling, except her daughters, who revealed mixed emotions. In a ward next door was another woman who had given birth to a girl. Only her mother was visiting and there was no smile on either of their faces.

Indian society views the perfect child as a boy, the imperfect child is a girl. She is a burden to her family as a child and, unless married, a social outcast. Social attitudes mean that girls do not get the education or training to enable them to be economically independent. The arguments put forward in favour of limiting the population of girl babies sound very familiar. In expressing his outrage at what is going on in his country, Professor Raj Sachar said, 'This type of population control could be something similar to Hitler trying to propagate the pure race by getting rid of all the Jews'. He went on further to say that Indian law permitted abortion, which he thought was right, but that the selective killing of foetuses was something 'No civilized society can accept'. Dr Sachar was very clear that what was needed to stop the practice was a change in social attitudes, stating very firmly 'It is only society that can stop it'.

Dr Raj Sachar gives, in fact, a way into opening up a public debate on the issues involved in prenatal testing. For women in Britain, there has been an understandable reluctance to open up this debate. The struggle for the right of women to choose whether or not to have an abortion is an ongoing one. Since 1967, when the Abortion Act was passed, women have had to be ever-vigilant in protecting their right to choose. Women fear that to question this right in any way is to open up the floodgate to the moral Right who are waiting in the wings to seize on any possible waivering in the ethical climate to try to change the law and restrict a woman's right to choose.

In all this debate, the terminology used is interesting. 'Termination' is what is offered women whose foetuses are found to have an abnormality. Termination is a much gentler word, reflecting the social respectability of what is on offer. 'Abortion' is a much more loaded term, reflecting a different, more censorious set of social attitudes. In this loaded linguistic debate, women have to assert the right to choose. They have to argue for the right to make an informed choice, including the right, without pressure or coercion, to choose whether or not to be tested. They should also have the right, if they choose to be tested, to make a decision on the results of the test. Informed consent is consent given on the basis of having information, not consent given prior to having information, as is now expected of many women agreeing to be tested. They have a right to have information given to them in neutral, non-directional language. Given that, in the present climate, those giving information have clearly *non-neutral* views, women should be given information from different sources, reflecting different attitudes. These rights should form part of any prenatal testing programme in every antenatal clinic.

The problem, of course, is not peculiar to antenatal clinics. The decision is not a clinical one, but one about social attitudes. It is about how our society values different groups of people. The pressure on a woman to choose one way or another comes not just from those health professionals informing and advising her. There is wider social pressure and it is this that I sensed all those years ago. *Choosing* to bring a Down's Syndrome child into this world could, I sensed, be seen as an irresponsible act, undeserving of support. In the recent research work by Theresa Marteau, she has found that women do not just sense, but actually *feel* 'guilty' for proceeding with a pregnancy in the knowledge that they will give birth to a child with a disability. 'Given the option', she writes, 'of prenatal diagnosis and abortion of affected foetuses, some parents feel that to produce a child with a potentially diagnosable handicap is to be blame-worthy for that child's birth. Indeed in the US some disabled children, including some with Down's Syndrome, have been awarded damages for wrongful life, on the basis that their disability should have been diagnosed before their birth and they should have been aborted'.

Prenatal screening, the tool that should enable women to *make* choices, is, in fact, in its practice, *limiting* choices. The pressures on women limiting their choices were expressed eloquently by Dr Robyn Rowland, who commented in an article in *the Guardian* that, 'Birth, pregnancy and now conception are largely in the hands of masculine medical science. Increasingly pressure is placed upon women to create the perfect product'. In this climate she asks, 'How do women say no to the use of technology? Will they be punished if they refuse to use it? Will any woman be able to conceive and move through the stages of pregnancy and birth without intervention? More and more, it becomes difficult for women to give birth and nurture the imperfect child. Will it be in the future that fewer and fewer social supports go to these women who should have done something to avoid it in the first place?' There is, indeed, an urgent need for public debate on these issues.

5 / The family

> The terrible pain of the tearing was quickly overtaken by the appearance of Jessie's head followed by the wonderful moment when her whole body was finally delivered. Straightaway she was laid down on my tummy. She wriggled and cried and seemed even at the moment of birth, vibrant. She looked normal. She was alive. I put her to the breast and she sucked. Effortlessly she knew what to do. I was amazed. Ed and I took turns in holding her and drinking the cups of tea they had brought for us.

That moment of Jessie's birth was one of true joy. I have told her many times that, for me, her first cry was the greatest and most moving sound I have ever heard. It was the cry of life. Ed and I knew from that sound that we were in the presence of a new life force, determinedly imprinting her individual personality on all around. She, at that moment, was launching out into life with new experiences ahead of her. We were starting a new life with her with memories.

These memories informed our first reaction and continue to inform our parenting of her 16 years later. All parents are overjoyed by the birth of a normal, healthy baby, and all parents are overawed by the sense of the preciousness of this new, tiny, human life they have created. Our sense of joy and relief were immediately understandable to all around. Our sense of her preciousness, even from the first moment of holding her, could only be appreciated by others who have experienced the death of a child. It was and is this sense of preciousness that has been at the core of our relationship with her. For Jessie, preciousness has been a burden she has carried since birth and is one that, at times, she wishes she could be free from.

I have learned over the years, and continue to learn, just how much the death of a child informs and affects all members of the family and the interrelationships of the family thereafter. I wrote the first draft of *Will, My Son* when Jessie was about two. The timing was significant. I felt I had come through the initial emotional and physical struggles of her early infancy. Although declared 'normal' by the paediatrician who checked her the day after she was born, I spent the first two years watching and waiting to see if she would see, hear, walk and talk. I did not feel totally reassured that Jessie was normal until she visibly demonstrated that she was. Fortunately, she was a quick learner, eager to be mobile and articulate.

Reflecting my concern, I did not even begin to resume any work until she was a year old and, then, very tentatively, I worked part time. Before Will's birth, I had planned how I would combine a baby and writing a history book. Not one word was written until a long time after his death. With Jessie, I did not plan anything. I stayed at home – not because I think mother's should be at home full time, but because I needed to be at home. That time at home, settling in with her, was, I know, beneficial for me and my emotional well-being. The call from a colleague, asking if I would like to do some part-time teaching at The National Film School came at the right moment. I was beginning to feel a need to get out of the home. The first few days I worked, I was physically out of the home, but, mentally, I did not leave it. I fretted and worried about Jessie all the time. However, slowly I found that I could go to work and an hour or two would pass without me worrying. Slowly the worrying lessened and my enjoyment in work increased. I found, like other mothers, that if you are confident in the child care arrangements and your child is healthy and happy, then you limit the worry level you take in your head to work to a manageable level. By the time Jessie was two, I felt I had, with a good wind, this ability. By the time I wrote the second draft of *Will, My Son*, I had even, on a freelance contract, returned to a little documentary film directing.

With hindsight, I realize that I clearly, optimistically thought life had settled down to the normal problems of a working mother and that I could balance my life between work and motherhood without memories undercutting my equilibrium. How wrong I was. To anyone who pauses to reflect a moment, it must be obvious that the death of a child must have a profound affect on how one parents any others. However, all to often, the obvious can pass us by. Caught up in the day-to-day parenting of a child, it is all too easy to be unaware of the underlying emotional agenda. When the experience of the death of one child is informing this emotional agenda, recognizing it is even harder. This is not helped by the prevailing social attitude that having a new baby somehow replaces the dead one. In *Will, My Son* I wrote:

> In fact I think the conventional advice given to people by doctors and lay people alike that after the death of one child they should 'have another as quickly as possible' is irresponsible. It is advice that considers the parents but not the child-to-be. Another child should start life as a new individual and not under pressure to replace a dead child. That advice implies that you can *replace* a dead child, that you can replace people. But people are not replaceable as human beings.

Progress has been made in recognizing that a mourning period is needed following the death of one child before embarking on the creation of another. However, even those who recognize that such a period is required give the implicit message that having 'dealt' with your grief, you can and should be able to move on and put the experience behind you. Some years after writing *Will, My Son* I made a television programme called *Whatever It Takes* on bereavement. I read quite a lot and talked to many people about the subject at the time, but in neither personal autobiographical material nor in the material, written by professionals working in the field of bereavement counselling, did I find anything about the long-term effects of the death of one child on the parenting of another. Had I done so, it might have alerted me to my own patterns of behaviour. A reflection of my own lack of awareness was that participating in *Whatever It Takes* was a mother who had also experienced the death of a young child. At the time of making the programme, her other children were young adults. Although we talked about many aspects of bereavement, I never asked her about how it had affected her mothering of her other children. I remained aware only of the most obvious ways in which the death of Will informed my treatment of and relationship with Jessie.

One of the obvious problems I recognized and continue to recognize is my heightened fears that are triggered whenever Jessie has a serious illness.

> The first time she was ill we both found particularly difficult. She had quite a severe attack of bronchitis and just as she was beginning to get better she started vomiting which frightened both of us. I remember Ed just bursting into tears and I knew the tears were a sudden welling up to the surface of memories and fears. From time to time if Jessie is ill or has a fall I get a tight sick feeling in the pit of my stomach, but mostly I feel I can lead a normal life and let her lead a normal life.

That sick feeling in the pit of my stomach has returned over the years to remind me of how close to the surface my terror is. I have not learned to deal with her illnesses philosophically.

Whooping cough was, for me, the worst. It started as a cold and cough in Canada. Flying back, Jessie coughed through the whole journey. The poor woman next to us, who did not have a quiet, restful flight, at one point suggested that Jessie might have whooping cough. 'Just a touch of bronchitis', I said confidently. When Jessie had finished the course of antibiotics the doctor prescribed for her 'touch of bronchitis', she was still coughing. It was then that the doctor suggested it might be whooping cough. Jessie had not been vaccinated for whooping cough as we had been advised against it, on the basis of family history. As an epidemic was in full swing, I began to suspect that the doctor might be right. It was some weeks after the first coughing that she started whooping. When she did, her whole little body would go into spasm. If she was standing, she would suddenly double over with her bottom up and whoop and gasp. One evening, while in a whooping spasm, she began to go blue. I had seen a blue child before - Will.

Our awareness that Will had problems with his heart began with a summer cold. Having been advised to take any cold seriously, I phoned the Home Care Unit with whom Will was registered and the Doctor, as always, promptly visited me at home. After examining Will, she prescribed antibiotics and digitalis. The latter, she gently explained, was a heart stimulant. Later that day, I drove down to my parents house to stay with them.

> Soon after arriving I began to get quite frightened. Will was breathing with difficulty. At one point my mother had him sitting on her knee and he began to go blue. For some reason she laid him on his back. I shouted at her 'sit him up, sit him up'. She did so and he returned to his normal colour. That night was a long and frightening one. I stayed up with him almost all night. He slept fitfully and I tried to keep him, whilst sleeping, with his head slightly raised, but he would keep sliding down flat onto his back, get into breathing difficulties, begin to go blue and would have to be rescued.

To see another child of mine, Jessie, go blue was to touch on my deepest fears. Ed was still in Canada at the time, but, fortunately, a close friend of mine, Jennifer, was staying with me. She gave me support, cups of coffee and her own, inimitable humour. That night is one that neither she nor I have forgotten for, throughout the night, Jessie had more spasms that turned her blue. It was the low moment of whooping cough and, although Jessie continued to cough for a long time after, she never again turned that terrifying, unnatural colour. Needless to say, for the months Jessie was ill my work was put on one side.

The following year was the year of scarlet fever. Jessie had been off school for a day, but, as she appeared to have nothing serious, I agreed to let her go on a school trip the following day. Having offered to help out, I knew that I would be there if she wasn't well. Outside Buckingham Palace, I became aware she was not well. By the time we reached the Tower of London, I knew she had a temperature. The following day, I went to work and Ed stayed at home with her. By this time, we were worried and had called the doctor. Late in the morning, I phoned home to check if the doctor had called. 'Scarlet fever', Ed said. My heart sank. Visions of dying Victorians flashed through my mind. My first reaction was to forget that we are living in the twentieth century and not in nineteenth century literature. I was quickly brought up to date when I got home and was reassured that with modern antibiotics scarlet fever, or more importantly the complications that ensue from the disease, can largely be controlled. For about four days, Jessie lay on the sofa, a bright red, miserable child, which worried rather than frightened me. After that, recovery was quick and scarlet fever was to mark the last of her childhood illnesses.

For many years, Jessie was remarkably healthy. She barely had to have a day off school. The terrors of her illnesses were slowly becoming memories. Then, a few days before the autumn half term, when she was 14, she went down with what I thought was flu. At the end of the week, she seemed much better, so I thought it all right for her to go up and spend the weekend with my niece in Leeds. It was a long-planned visit. When I went to pick Jessie up at King Cross after the weekend, she was in tears and I could see that the glands in her neck were very swollen. The doctor examined Jessie and ruled out mumps, but suspected glandular fever. A blood test was requested, which was done that day by the nurse. Reassuringly, the nurse told us, 'We've done a lot of these recently, but they've all been negative'. I went home with no serious worry in my mind that Jessie's illness was anything more than an extended bout of flu, exacerbated by the fact that I had allowed her to go to Leeds for the weekend when, clearly, she hadn't fully recovered.

On the Friday morning, I left to go to Devon for the weekend. I had been invited to the eightieth birthday party of one of my uncles. Ed was with Jessie and I had left instructions that he was to phone the doctor's surgery for the results of her blood test, which were due in that day. In the evening, I phoned home. Ed told me that he had phoned the surgery and had been told by the receptionist that the results were through, but she couldn't communicate them directly to him, that he would have to make an appointment for us to see a doctor. An appointment had been made for Monday. I flipped, 'What do you mean she wouldn't tell you the results? Didn't you insist on talking to a doctor? Didn't you make a fuss? Didn't you go down to the surgery and demand the results'? I tiraded down the phone, exasperated by Ed's meekness in the face of the classic tyrannical surgery receptionist – a class of their own in my experience. I went on with my tirade,

'You do realize, don't you, that the results must show something is wrong with her. If it was negative *she'd* have told you. That is how the system works'. I had had considerably more experience of the system than Ed. Ed didn't seem to feel the fear or the urgency. 'Jessie seems all right. Just a bit tired', he said. I put down the phone and went into panic.

Doctors are a cause of high stress. Indeed, sometimes I think doctors contribute to stress-related illnesses. My doctor certainly caused me a huge amount of worry and stress that weekend. I kept thinking, the blood test has revealed something is wrong with her, something the receptionist cannot communicate over the phone, something only a doctor can tell us. It has to be serious. As the weekend wore on, in my mind, whatever it was she had got more and more serious. Doctors must know that to tell parents a blood test has revealed something is wrong with a child and then leave these parents for almost three days to find out exactly what is wrong with their child is a form of mental cruelty. One can only assume that the doctors themselves have never stopped to think of the emotional implications of their procedures. If they did they would change these procedures.

When we finally got to see a doctor with Jessie, we were told that the blood test revealed that she did, indeed, have glandular fever. Having a diagnosis was a huge relief. Glandular fever, which I had had in my early twenties, was, I knew, a long, drawn-out, demoralizing illness, but not life-threatening. I went home feeling much better and back to the 'I can cope' mode. In fact, I found dealing with the months of her illness much harder than I anticipated. It demoralized her and me. I had no work at the time and found it difficult to seriously motivate myself to look. I realized then just how much I am still on an emotional edge around her when she is ill. After the diagnosis, I had no more sleepless nights conjuring up the worst. I did not have to deal with the immediate terror of a child that had turned blue, but I did live through the months of her illness never quite relaxed and never quite at ease. Throughout Jessie's childhood people have said reassuringly, 'Don't worry, kids get through things, kids are tough' and I just smile. Inside I know that one kid didn't get through.

My lack of calm in the face of Jessie's serious illnesses is something other people have been and are very understanding about. For Jessie, too, it is perhaps the most acceptable and understandable aspect of our protectiveness of her. The pervasive protectiveness that informs our parenting of her is something she finds much harder to accept. Recently I read out to Jessie the following sentence from *Will, My Son*:

> Although we were, and still are, undoubtedly more protective of Jessie than many parents are of their children I think we manage most of the time to behave and react in a reasonably balanced way.

She laughed and said, 'You got that wrong, didn't you?' 'Yes', I confirmed, 'I got it very wrong.' This conversation was one of many similar ones we have had over the past year. It was Jessie that catapulted me into having to confront the oppressive effect our protectiveness, mine in particular, was having on her as she emerges, through adolescence, from childhood to womanhood.

This realization happened on a Thursday evening in November. Untypically, I got home from work after Ed. He greeted me as I came in through the door with a worried look on his face. I can't remember his exact words - something about Jessie's not here, she's gone. I didn't understand. He then showed me a note she had left for us. I went cold as I read it. It was short and stated 'I have run away'. She had then written. 'For once in your life, don't worry about me. I will go somewhere safe' and ended by saying, 'I love you'. Ed told me he had already phoned all her friends whose numbers we had. None of them knew anything about it or where she was. We kept calling her friends and calling back. Two came round to see us, but we could glean nothing. Soon after midnight, we got a call from a friend's house to say she was there, but she didn't want to see us. Ed went to the house. Jessie was adamant she didn't want to see us. Ed returned. For us, and, I am sure, for her, too, it was a long miserable night. We were all hurting. The following morning we phoned her. Ed talked to her briefly and then I talked to her. My calm broke. She could hear me crying down the phone. She said she would see us that evening, but that she wanted the day to herself. We respected her wishes.

In some kind of numbed, shocked state I went to work. I knew that if I stayed at home I would find it very hard not to try and see her, knowing she was but a few streets away. On my way to work, I stopped at the bank to cash a cheque. I walked in, took out my cheque book and glanced at the date. It was 20 November – the anniversary of Will's death. I fled from the bank in tears. I got in the car and sat weeping. Will was dead and Jessie had run away, was some place else and didn't want to see me. I felt as though I had lost two children. I felt bereaved.

At the time, the two experiences combining on one day just made the hurt even greater. Later, it was to be the key to helping me understand the emotional pressures I put on to Jessie and from which she felt she had to liberate herself. Had the dates *not* coincided, I might have never realized that what underlay my difficulties in dealing with Jessie breaking away from us and her home was that I feared it would be like another bereavement. It was a realization that came as a shock to me. Although over the years I have read a considerable amount about bereavement, nothing had forewarned or prepared me for the emotions that would be triggered by my daughter beginning the normal and healthy process of breaking away.

Talking to friends about my feelings, they have responded by saying, 'Well, it *is* a sort of bereavement', and I have replied very firmly, 'No, it is not'. The difference is absolute. When one is bereaved, hope is gone. What we are going through is change. In that there is a sense of loss. The childhood years are over. Jessie is in the middle of her rites of passage from childhood to womanhood. Like many other parents of teenagers, this means negotiating and renegotiating with her her freedom of movement. In this we are trying to achieve the delicate balance between allowing her to find her feet in the world and ensuring her safety while she does it. We have to be with her through this transition and, hopefully, emerge from it as adults with a new relationship. There is a whole new future before us.

Jessie running away came as a bolt out of the blue to us and our friends, to her friends and to her teachers. I remember Jessie telling me of the absolute surprise of her form tutor when she told her of the reason for her absence from school. Jessie had the same form tutor for four years, so she knew her well and we deeply appreciated that she was someone in whom Jessie could confide. The support and understanding by the school both of her and of us was a very important element in helping us all. Recognizing our history was also important for all concerned in understanding what was going on underneath. To others and to ourselves we appeared to be reasonable parents who were not unduly protective or restrictive. Some parents, we knew, were more lenient with their children, allowing them a freer rein to go out, stay out and not report back on their movements. Others, we knew, were stricter. Outsiders only saw the appearance of us as caring parents. They were unaware of the subtle pressures that children, with their hypersensitive antennae, pick up from their parents. It was these subtle pressures that Jessie had felt all her life. She didn't know how to articulate her feelings of oppression. At 15, the only way she felt she could send out a distress signal that all was not well was to run away.

That Friday evening, she came home, and we had the first of many conversations. The core of her angst was that she felt oppressed. 'I feel', she said, 'the burden of preciousness.' She went on to elaborate on this: 'I mean, I can't even cross the road without feeling I've got to be careful because, if anything happened to me . . .' She didn't have to finish the sentence. Another time she said, 'I feel as though all your hopes and happiness is invested in me'. In many different ways, she was saying, 'get off my back, give me space, let go'. We knew, myself in particular, that we had burdened her with preciousness. It was Ed and I, we knew, who had to change, but how?

We can, at one level, with a truth she recognized, reassure her that all our hopes and our happiness are *not* invested in her. We have our relationship with each other in which much of our mutual happiness is invested. She knows that we both have aspirations relating to our work, too. In the past, I remember saying to various people, 'It's lucky for Jessie that my work is very important to me. If I didn't have hopes and aspirations to write and make films (some of which come to fruition), the poor child would be the focus all my energies and dreams'. This, I knew, would be an unbearable pressure and burden for her.

Unfortunately, prior to her running away, I had had over a year of barely working, which was not a result of my choosing not to work, it simply happened that way. However, Jessie knew that my failure to get work was a source of unhappiness to me. I also knew that it bugged her having me round the house most of the time. She, like me, although very sociable, also loves time and space in the house on her own. This desire was something I could easily appreciate and I try to give it to her. In other ways, we realize that we have to reassure Jessie that we could find happiness in other aspects of our lives, though we did say to her that she had to give us time to change. After 15 years of focusing our lives on our child, we, like other parents with teenage children, are facing the realization that we are entering a new phase of life. It is one in which our child is slowly taking less and less of a central role in our day-to-day routines. Changing for us is a slow process, but we are aware that it is important for us and for her that we do make this change. For Jessie, change is happening at high speed. In every stage of her development we, as parents, have been running fast to keep up.

At the deepest level, reassuring her that a central pillar of our happiness is not invested in her is impossible. All parents live emotionally on the edge in their fear that their child may die before them. It is the deepest fear of parents. When Jessie used the words 'all your happiness is invested in me', there was an immediate echo in my head – an echo of an inscription on an eighteenth-century gravestone to a nine-year-old girl, Penelope Boothby. On it is written, 'The unfortunate parents ventured their all on this frail bark and the wreck was total'. There is no way I can honestly say to Jessie that I have no fear that 'the wreck' would not be 'total' if she were to die. Having survived the death of one child, I feel that I should draw strength from the knowledge that survival is possible. It is more than just possible, for I know that my life since Will's death has been rich; there have been many, many things over these years that have given me great happiness. One of the things that has made that life immeasurably richer has been Jessie. One line I wrote in *Will, My Son* that is as true today as it was when I wrote it is, 'She is a great source of happiness to Ed and me'.

My parenting of Jessie has been informed not only by Will's death, but also by the fact that he was Down's Syndrome. When pregnant with Jessie, my only wish was that she should be a normal, healthy child. I vowed that I would take joy merely in that fact. I vowed I would not expect her to fulfil any expectation that I might consciously or unconsciously have of her. We had been made sharply aware of how many unconscious dreams one has for one's child by the diagnosis that our first born was Down's Syndrome. I return once more to a passage from *Will, My Son* because it captures this natural tendency so absolutely:

> To have to come to terms with the fact that one's own flesh and blood, grown in one's own womb, is not normal is to have to come to terms with many things within oneself. It is an enormously humbling experience. In one stroke all those conscious and subconscious fantasies parents have for their children were knocked to the ground. Whilst Will was still in the incubator, before we knew of his mongolism, I remember Ed looking at one of his tiny feet and joking about how that might be the foot which scored the winning goal for Arsenal in a cup final twenty odd years hence. It was the kind of comment half joking, half fanciful, part wishing, that parents make, particularly of tiny babies. In the first few weeks after we knew about Will's handicap it was the kind of comment we did not make. We were painfully aware of all the things he definitely would not do. It left little room for us to have fantasies about greatness and glory.

Although I have never had conscious fantasies about Jessie achieving greatness and glory and have no conscious ambition for her that I expect her to fulfil, I know that I have expectations. It is hard sometimes to remember that vow I made to just take joy in her being when the pressure is on. This pressure comes partly from external sources - other people and partly from an internal desire to see one's child flourish and achieve. Other parents have a superb ability to sing the praises of their own little wonder, thereby trying to boost their own confidence as a parent and undermine yours. I have certainly been sensitive to such pressures. What is hardest of all, though, is trying to achieve a balance between encouragement that one hopes is positive and pressure that, ultimately, is negative.

What I do know is that 'achievements' are important, but they are only one of the rewards of life. I know that at a deep level. I understood absolutely, when reading in *Living In The Real World* the feelings of one mother when she described her changed perspective, which had been brought about by having a Down's Syndrome son: 'Hamish has brought it home to us', she said, 'I must admit the down-to-earth joy of living and being with one another and enjoying one another is more important. Because nothing is taken for granted, you know: every day with Hamish is precious, because life is not just taken for granted. When Hamish was one year old, they told me he didn't need heart surgery – that to me was pure joy. I thought, *anything*, I don't care what you're capable of or what you're not capable of, that's all right because he doesn't need heart surgery, and to me that's how it stands. I really do appreciate everything about him, and whatever he can achieve is great'.

When we say that all we want for Jessie is that she is healthy and happy, it is not a trite cliché. That is the baseline for us; everything else is a bonus. There are times when I have listened to parents talking about whether or not their child gets their GCSE's, A levels, university degrees as though it is more important than anything else in the world. Of course I am concerned about Jessie's exams and how she will do in them – I was proud and delighted by her GCSE achievements – but my happiness is not invested in the results alone. It was with total disbelief that I heard of a mother who was in floods of tears because her son had failed to get a first-class degree and, thus, in her eyes, was a failure. We had learned with Will to take pleasure in all his achievements. Over the years, we have also taken great pleasure in watching Jessie develop her talents, which are many, but we know, and hope she knows, that our love is not *conditional* on her achieving.

Jessie's place in the family is seen in different ways by her and by us. Jessie sees herself as an only child. This is hardly surprising as this has been her experience. For us, she is our second child. These differing perspectives and experiences have created curious tensions. Sometimes I wonder if they would have been resolved, or certainly lessened, had we had more children. We did not plan to only have Jessie; neither did we plan to have more. As things turned out, we did not have any more. Shortly after Jessie was born, Ed, high on being a father again, suggested we quickly try to conceive another. I, tired and body battered from giving birth, said I would rather wait a while to give me a chance to get back to mental and physical working order. When I had recovered from the birth and breastfeeding, I did, from time to time, contemplate having another child. Ed, by this time, had lost the strong urge to have another child, though I knew that, had I really wanted to go ahead, he would have supported the idea. However, whenever I seriously thought of having another child, my fear that something would go wrong took hold. With Jessie, my desire to have another baby had been so great it somehow drove me forward during pregnancy. Once Jessie was firmly placed in my life, this desire was greatly diminished. The fear took over, weighting the scales against having another child; I could not bring myself to even try to conceive.

Others, still in their fertile years, respond to the death of one child differently. Some go on and have more, sometimes several more children. Others cannot open themselves to the possibility of such pain again. For me, the main reason I did not have another child after Jessie was the fear of having another child with a disability, one who might be much more severely disabled than Will. There have been times when I have felt I should have fought this fear. Although many children are 'only children', society still views the normal family unit as one in which there are, or should be, at least two children. As a parent of an only child, you feel guilty that you are depriving them of siblings. When your child is sitting on the beach lonely, and with no one to play with; when your child is about the only one in the class not to put their hand up to the question 'who has got brothers and sisters?'; when you know they have no one to gang up with in solidarity against unreasonable parents, you feel responsible for their isolation. Jessie did once ask on Christmas Eve for a brother or sister for Christmas, but most of the time she is aware of the benefits of being an only child. These are not what her friends assume them to be - material benefits - but the benefits of being secure in the knowledge that our love is for her and her

The family / 141

alone. There are no siblings to fight for attention or love. Yet, it is not quite as simple as that. She knows that she had a brother, someone we loved very deeply and whose death we still mourn.

From as young as she can remember she has known she had a brother. A photograph of him hangs in a silver frame on the wall in our sitting room. I cannot remember consciously telling her about him; she just assimilated this from our conversations and from the photo of Will. The concept of death was one she grasped young. The non-existence of her brother made very real for her the meaning of death, though there were a few confusions on the way to understanding. When she was quite small, we took her to the gardens at the crematorium to visit Will's small commemorative plaque. Afterwards, walking around, looking at other plaques, Jessie, who was old enough to decipher numbers but not old enough to understand their meaning, looked at the dates on the plaques and asked 'Are they the dead people's phone numbers?' We could not help but smile a bitter-sweet smile.

It was with a similar smile, I remember, that I responded another time. I was outside the sitting room door and heard her, when quite small, explaining that the baby in the photo was her brother. Another time, I was driving her and a friend somewhere. They were in the back, talking, and, at some point in their conversation, I heard Jessie explaining to her friend that she had had a brother who had died before she was born.

For me, I needed no more than she should claim him. I remember one anniversary of his death and Jessie, sensitive to others, detected my mood of sadness. I told her why I was feeling sad. She said, 'I know I ought to feel sad, but I don't. I never knew him. I can't feel sad about someone I never knew'. I reassured her that she was not expected to feel sad, indeed, she couldn't possibly feel something for someone she had never known. There was, I told her, absolutely nothing wrong or hard-hearted about her absence of feeling. All that she should understand was that *I* felt sad.

My sadness then and at other times is a reminder to her of her second child status. There have been a few times over the years when I think that she has felt threatened by the presence of Will in our memories. It is a chink in the security of her only child view. There is an element of normal sibling jealousy in this. She has, once or twice, when feeling threatened, indirectly asked, 'Why is Will written about, talked about and has his photo on the wall?' 'Because', I tell her, 'I have you here with me. I can see you, touch you, hear you and, besides, there are far more photos of you around the house than there are of Will.' This interaction has only happened once or twice, but it has been enough to make me realize that she needs the reassurance that our love for her is not in any way diminished by the fact that we loved Will.

E D

I fear the effect it will have on my relationship with Ed.

I wrote this when I was about five months' pregnant with Will. My fears, at that time, were general. They were based on the knowledge that 'something happened' to people after the birth of a child and that 'something' seemed to primarily happen to women. Their lives changed. I was apprehensive as to whether or not our relationship could be maintained, let alone flourish, under such change. The experience of Will did have a profound effect on my relationship with Ed in ways that I could neither have anticipated nor even have comprehended before his birth.

The problem, of course, is that, until you have a baby, there is absolutely no way anyone can communicate to you just how much the experience will change you. For women without children, as I was, motherhood appears to be primarily a problem of economics, time and ties. For women with a child, it is about having your whole being changed. The time and ties are a question of organization. The deep emotional change in human values that women undergo in the act of giving birth is, from all I have read, heard and experienced, uncommunicable. There is a huge divide between women who do have children and women who don't. There is also a deep tension in this divide. To me, although I think it should be talked about by women in general, this divide is much more comprehensible than the divide between mothers and fathers.

Women, however, have found it much more comfortable to talk and write about this latter gender divide. At its extreme, the divide is revealed by the number of fathers who walk out on their children. For parents who remain together, the divide is usually obvious from the daily patterns of their lives. Fatherhood means little change for the majority. This is evident not just in their day-to-day lives, which, for most, undergo minimal change, but in what appears to be an unchanged emotional response to the world. Not surprisingly, mothers, who have undergone such profound change, cannot understand how fathers, the father of their child no less, have not. Although both parents may well deeply love the child (or children), this love, as a living experience, means different things to fathers and mothers. At least, one can only draw this conclusion from the evidence.

This different emotional response to parenting was something I was completely unprepared for. I had assumed that having a child would mean we would have to reorganize our lives. In this reorganization I assumed that an equality would continue, after the interruption of maternity leave, and that, somehow, we would share the responsibilities of earning the family wage and of looking after our child equally. None of this took on board our feelings. Events overtook all these assumptions. I was suddenly propelled by the situation, and my emotional response to it, into becoming a full-time mother.

Throughout the nine months of Will's life, Ed got up and went to work. He took short periods off work at different times to be with me and to deal with his own emotional needs. I don't think it ever entered his head that he might do otherwise. Work and earning a living were what he unquestioningly did and wanted to do. There were a few interruptions to work during that year. Paternity leave was not then a right, but he did take, as holiday, the equivalent. We had a short summer holiday all together and Ed took time off work to be with me when Will had heart surgery and after Will's death. It was not just that Ed *assumed* that his daily life would go on as normal, it *did* go on as normal, with a few minor changes. These changes affected our relationship much in the same way any first baby affects a couple. We were unable to go out together unless we had a babysitter. We rarely did get a babysitter as I was very reluctant to leave Will, particularly after his heart defect had been diagnosed, with anyone in whom I did not have absolute confidence. On the other hand, Will was such a good baby he was no trouble if he accompanied us. We could take him with us to friends for the evening and know that he would not disrupt our evening. At home, Ed would change and bath Will, feed him and play with him. He would wash nappies and cook meals. He loved Will, of that there was no doubt.

I knew, too, that his love was for Will as he was - a Down's Syndrome child. Our emotional responses to the news of his disability were the same. We took strength and comfort from each other. After we had been told that he had Down's Syndrome:

> Ed spent the whole week at home and we barely parted from each other's company. We developed a sensitivity to each other's moods. One would sense when the other was needing reassurance or just a hug and usefully one was normally feeling strong when the other was weak.

For both of us, we were facing our own sense of failure - failure to produce a normal child. The future, we both felt, was daunting, but we were at one in facing it. It was me, however, that dealt with the practical realities of starting out on this future with our child.

For nine months, my life was, in every way, involved with Will. I breastfed him throughout. From the age of six months, I had started to wean him, and, by nine months, he was down to a token night-time breastfeed. My days, too, were filled with looking after him. In the practicalities of life with a small baby, my experiences were not that much different from most other mothers. Throughout, though, it was I, not Ed, who was in the front line when dealing with both Will's disability and his physical problems. I was the one who pursued information about Down's Syndrome, phoning people up, looking for literature and arranging for us to see people. I was also the one who stayed in hospital with Will. Of that, however, Ed was offered little choice. In the mid-seventies, staying in hospital with one's child was not expected. Hospitals, by then, had improved from the days when parents were strictly restricted to visiting hours, but parents 'hanging around' all day and night was not accepted practice. Little provision was made for it and the little there was, was based on the assumption that only mothers would stay overnight. However, there was choice in taking Will to see doctors and consultants. It was I who did this, though, and had to report back to Ed the latest piece of bad news. It was not that Ed refused to come with us; a more complicated interpersonal dynamic was set up. I fronted up mostly, not just to the wider world, but also to Ed, with my well-developed public 'I can cope' mode. This made it easy for Ed to leave me to cope. I would then feel resentful that he had left me to cope on my own. For me, to ask for support is hard. For Ed, to offer support is hard. Ed says, 'You only have to ask'. I say, 'Why do I have to ask?' For many women, and men, this probably sounds very familiar.

One incident illustrates this scenario. Shortly after we had had the first indication that something was wrong with Will's heart, I had to take him to see a consultant.

> I told Ed it was not necessary for him to take time off work to come with me this time and that I could cope.
> . . .
> The consultant looked at Will, listened to his heart and then turned to me and said 'We'll have to admit him, he's in a state of heart failure'. No further explanation was given. I was shown into a neighbouring room and handed over to a nurse who was to arrange for his admission. The shock was terrible. For a long time I was left on my own sitting in the bare room, holding Will and feeling dazed. After finding out that it would be some time before Will was actually admitted I phoned Ed and in tears asked him to come to the hospital explaining briefly why. Ed came.

With hindsight, I should have asked Ed to come with me in the first place. Yet there is another part of me that cannot understand why, if your child is having to see a consultant because it is already known that there is something wrong with their heart, that you do not want to be there. I cannot understand how you cannot be there.

In this lack of understanding is the divide. One can talk about men's roles, the economic pressures, the burden of being the breadwinner and the fact that they are so often marginalized from the act of parenting, including being marginalized by mothers. One knows that our whole economic and social structure has been created to marginalize men from fathering. Yet, it is men who have created these structures - or have they. Is it chicken or egg? Did the structures lead to the marginalization of men or did men, marginal from childbirth, create these structures? Where in all the nature and nurture debates are their emotions?

In the emotional situation in which we found ourselves, Ed and I are little different from most other mothers and fathers. The only difference was in our particular circumstances. These circumstances both heightened the divide *and* brought us much more closely together. The tension between what we both feel is the divide between our emotional responses to parenting and the closeness that the experience of parenting has brought us has been central to our relationship.

Just as we were as one in our response to the knowledge of Will's Down's Syndrome, we were as one in our response to his death. Throughout his life, we had been together in affirming to the world that our son was loved and valued. Our emotions at his death were simple: we had lost the son we loved, we both grieved. I have heard of more than one father who has got up the day after his child's death and gone to work. Indeed, it was reported to me that the head of a department in the BBC said proudly to his troops that he had been back at work the day after his child died. He, in saying this, no doubt assumed that such an action would increase people's respect for him and his commitment to work. Clearly he did not realize that, for many in his audience, this piece of information *lost* him respect - respect as a sentient human being. I understand that getting up and going to work may be a survival mechanism for some. It is how, in their grief, they manage to go on. Everyone who is bereaved has to find their own ways of survival. It is also a reflection of the emotional place work has in men's lives that it can be used as a way of denying other emotions. However, to boast about it has to make one question the value system of that individual and of the society that has inculcated those values. My other reaction to this story was to think of his partner. How did she feel, left alone at home with her grief, while her husband went off to work? How has their relationship survived this divide?

At one level, grief is or can be shared – the level of support and understanding. Ed and I were together in our grief. The week between Will's death and the funeral, we spent together. Ed could not have got up and gone to work the day after Will's death, and he could not have left me alone. After the funeral, we went away for two weeks to put a little space and time between Will's death and having to start our lives again. This togetherness in the face of Will's death, both emotionally and physically, was, with hindsight, very important for the survival of our relationship.

However, on another level, grief, or, rather, the act of grieving, cannot be shared. In grief you are totally separate and alone. Ed and I could and did offer each other support and understanding and yet we knew that each was trapped in their own world of pain. Just as you do not feel the pain of someone else's pin prick, you do not feel the pain of someone else's grief. I could *observe* Ed's pain, but I could not feel it, and neither could he feel mine.

The most eloquent description of the separation brought about by grief I have read was written by Sean O'Casey. For fours years after the death of his son, Niall, Sean O'Casey kept a diary of his grief. O'Casey himself died in 1964 and this diary was not published until 1991, when his wife, Eileen, felt it should no longer remain private. In his entry for 28 September, 1957, O'Casey wrote, 'I am bright with those who come to see me, for it is not for them to be harassed with the sorrow inflicting me. I alone can enter with the terrible silence of my dead boy. Not even Eileen can come with me, for she, too, has to enter her own region of silence alone when she thinks of, and sorrows after our dead boy. She enters the terrible alone to share it with her beloved boy; enters silently when no one knows; as I do too, when no one knows, not even she, for neither of us tells the other; it is a secret and silent communion with the silence of our beloved, our dearly beloved son'.

It does not surprise me that the break-up rate of relationships following the death of a child is very high. When each is so isolated in their own efforts to survive emotionally as a person, it is very hard for the *relationship* to survive. The pursuit of survival takes different paths and these paths can end in a parting of the ways, even when neither guilt nor blame is involved. After Will's death, we were thrown back on each other as a couple. We were profoundly changed, struggling to survive as individuals *and* as a couple. Of course, none of this behaviour took the form of conscious decision making; we were in the realms of bare emotions. We each, individually, had to get up and go on and we each, individually, worked out our ways of doing this.

For Ed, getting up and going on was made easier by the fact that he had a full-time job that he had to go to. Also, he has always, then and now, invested most of himself in his pursuit of work. Work is his source of earning a living, of finding and affirming his identity, of most of his social relations (family excluded) and a major source of fulfilment in his life.

For me, getting up and going on was much more difficult. First, I had to *find* a job. I did have a book to write, but I knew that, at that point in time, I had to get out of the house. Going out to work on a TV pilot series was not a deeply fulfilling experience, though I was very grateful at the time to the person who, knowing my situation, got me the job. Writing my book, a history book, when I returned to it was rewarding, but I knew that it was no longer as important to me as it was when I was researching it prior to Will's birth. No work would have the same importance ever again. The time between the death of Will and the birth of Jessie was, for me, a case of lurching from one survival strategy to another. What held Ed and me together in those raw days was our love for each other and our unspoken understanding that each had to do what they had to do. At times, our behaviour may have seemed, indeed was at times, selfish and hurtful to the other. Survival behaviour is not always unselfish, loving and caring. The other bond we had was a deep desire to create another child together.

I naively thought that I would return to some emotional norm once Jessie was born. I do not remember consciously thinking about the effect her birth would have on Ed and me. We both assumed that Ed would go on working with a brief paternity leave interruption, although this was never discussed. For myself, I decided to plan nothing. With Will, all my carefully laid plans had been blown apart. This time, I decided to take childbirth and my emotional response to it stage by stage. Although I did, after about a year, return to work as a freelance, my work has always been intermittent. What I know, however, is that the value I put on my work is of a different order to that which Ed puts on his. It is not that my work is unimportant to me, that I am lukewarm about it or that I find it unsatisfying and unfulfilling, quite the opposite, but, since Jessie was born, she has taken centre stage in my life. Work has had to fit in with her in terms of my emotional commitment. This has been particularly difficult in my field of work – independent documentary film making – where getting work is dependent on the single-minded pursuit of this end. Having been commissioned to make a film, equally single-minded commitment to the film is also expected. Even though I have always been deeply committed to any film I have made, at the end of the day, it is, for me, 'only a film' and not to be confused with real life. Neither in the pursuit of my work, nor in its execution, could I follow a single-minded approach.

For Ed and me, the differences in our parenting of Jessie have not been in the emotions, but in the emotional commitment. From the moment of Jessie's birth, there has never been a shadow of doubt in my mind about Ed's love for Jessie. Before we knew that she was a girl as a result of amniocentesis, we both, first, hoped our child would be normal and healthy and, second, that the child would be a girl. We thought that if it was a girl, it would help us to make a new start with this new life. However, beyond these shared wishes, Ed particularly wanted a daughter, contrary to the assumed normal desire of fathers to have a son, so he was delighted to find that our child was a girl. He has delighted in having a daughter ever since. The divide for us has not been one of either of us loving Jessie more or less, it has been one of how this love is expressed. It is in the emotional commitment, in the daily living expression of this commitment, that the divide in our response to having a child has been manifested itself. This emotional commitment is, from my observation and experience, where the divide between fathers and mothers lies. In this divide there is a gulf of understanding.

Nothing had prepared us for this gulf. We entered parenting equal, or as equal as men and women in our society can be. We had similar academic qualifications. We both had aspirations for achievement in and fulfilment through our work. Ed has never expected, in any way pressurized, me to stay at home and look after Jessie. Indeed, it has been the opposite. He has always encouraged me to work. I demanded equality and got it. We share the economic burden of supporting our family unit, though Ed feels the extra burden of needing to ensure his job security in the face of my job insecurity. He would argue that the 'neurosis' attached to ensuring one steady family income has led him to work harder and longer than perhaps he might otherwise have done. While he took on this extra burden, I felt, and feel, that I took on the prime responsibility for the well-being of the family unit. I didn't intellectually *choose* to take it on, but my emotional response to my child left me no option but to do so. It is a response that most mothers recognize. For me, however, it was greatly heightened by the death of Will. I had lost one child. I knew the value of human life and personal relationships. Everything else was and is secondary.

Ed, in investing so much of himself in his work, and myself, investing so much in Jessie, has meant that, often, each of us has felt neglected: Ed certainly felt Jessie was more important to me than he was; I certainly felt that his work almost always seemed to take priority over my or Jessie's needs. I felt that, through Will's death, I had learned so much about the real emotional baseline of life that I could not understand why Ed seemed to have learned so little. My life has been changed completely by birth, death and birth in a way that I feel Ed's has not.

Ed, like many men of his generation, is unsure of what is expected of him as a father. His father, it would appear, suffered no such confusion. He *knew* that his primary role was that of breadwinner and his wife's was that of mother and homemaker. We thought these roles should be redefined, but never really redefined them. How much our failure to do so was our own refusal to fight it out or the fact that we were caught in a particular period of time when attitudes, not practices, were changing, it is hard to assess. Although our domestic life, and the division of labour within it, has been different to that of our parents, when the emotional chips are down, the change has not been that great.

Reading the above, people may wonder why and how our relationship has survived. Relationships work for a number of reasons and we are no different to others in this respect. We share many things, from being tidy to our general ethical, political and social views. We have always had a close physical relationship. Being a couple has never meant, for us, doing everything together. Over the years we have always respected each other's need for separate friends and leisure activities. However, shared experiences have also been very important. Three years ago, we went as a family to Austin, Texas, for four months. Ed was invited to lecture on Western films for a semester at the University. Jessie and I went with him. She went to school there and I occupied myself with writing a book. For all of us, it was an important, shared experience that we thoroughly enjoyed. Another strength in our relationship is that we have been at one in all the major decisions relating to Jessie's upbringing. Indeed, we share much.

Part of what we share is our history. We have faced together the extremities of emotions: we have shared the joy of birth and stood together over the body of our dead son. We have held on to each other when neither of us were sure how each could hold on to themselves. We have been humbled by our feelings that, as individuals, and as a couple, we 'failed' to produce a normal child. We share our love of Jessie and our understanding of the vulnerability that our love of her engenders in each of us. We have a lot of history that is shared. In this history is also a lot of love for each other. There is a common wisdom that if you, as a couple, survive such experiences as the death of a child, then your relationship is much stronger. There is an element of truth in this assumption, but merely to say it is to grossly oversimplify the complicated emotions.

As Jessie grows up and, step by step, leaves us and home, Ed and I have to, equally, step by step, readjust to being a couple again. The last time we had to make this adjustment was when we were brutally forced back into coupledom following the death of Will. This time, after the initial trauma, we enter this new phase in our life more gently, but we carry into it our emotional histories and the effect that this history has had on our life. In his early fifties, Ed marches forward, in terms of achievement, through his work. Approaching fifty, I am not sure, what the future holds in career terms. This state of affairs, obviously, is partly about the different work we each chose to pursue.

My choice, that of an independent documentary film maker, was not, even without a child, an easy career choice. I do know, however, that most of the women in my industry who have been successful and reached, not the top, for that is still almost exclusively a male preserve, but the higher echelons, are without children. I also know that having children does not inhibit most men's career advancement. Had I been a father, pursuing the same career with the same skills as myself, the story would almost certainly have been very different. At the heart of this difference, once you scrape away the layers of discrimination against women, particularly in film and TV, is the difference of an emotional response to the importance and value of nurturing one human life. In particular, the life of one's child. Of course, this is not true for *every* father and *every* mother, but it is true for many and it is true for me. True for me, also, as it is for all the other mothers I have talked to, is that our decision to make an emotional commitment to our children our first priority is one none of us have any regrets about.

In day-to-day terms, the tensions between Ed and me over 'the divide' recede as Jessie becomes more independent. It also lessens because her needs are ones that we can both meet equally without causing major interruptions in our lives: Jessie needs love, guidance, advice and money! She does not need anyone to babysit her, pick her up from school or look after her in the holidays. For me, of course, this means a major change in my life, while for Ed it means that he can both fulfil his obligations and commitments to work *and* be a good and loving father without conflict.

As the tensions recede, so do the feelings that this tension gave rise to. For me, I realize that the only way forward is to accept that parenting meant different things for each of us. This difference emanated from our emotional responses. These responses have informed our life patterns. With the demands of active parenting (one is always a parent emotionally) receding in terms of our daily lives, we have to work out a new life pattern with each other. I am reluctant to predict the future. I do not assume that, because of the past, our relationship will make it through the future. Ed and I never married and never promised 'til death do us part'. But my love for him and all that we have experienced together in the past makes me want to go forward into the future with him by my side.

6 / Grief

What though the radiance which was once so bright
Be now for ever taken from my sight
Though nothing can bring back the hour
Of splendour in the grass, of glory in the flower;
We will grieve not, rather find
Strength in what remains behind;
In the primal sympathy
Which having been must ever be;
In the soothing thoughts that spring
Out of human suffering;
In the faith that looks through death,
In years that bring the philosophic mind . . .

Thanks to the human heart by which we live,
Thanks to its tenderness, its joys, and fears,
To me the meanest flower that blows can give
Thoughts that do often lie too deep for tears.

This extract from Wordsworth's *Ode on Intimations of Immortality from Recollections of Early Childhood* we had read at Will's funeral. Over the years, I have found 'strength in what remains behind', but I have grieved and still grieve. I live with 'Thoughts that do often lie too deep for tears'.

The need for grief to be recognized was something I felt strongly about when writing *Will, My Son*. In writing of my grief, I was speaking out against the dominant attitude that, after an accepted mourning period of, at most, a few weeks, one should get on with one's life. This attitude serves the interests of, and emotionally protects, the non-bereaved, not the bereaved. It leaves the bereaved isolated, in pain and unsure of their own mental stability. A few months after Will's death, I had resumed what, to an observer, might appear a normal life. My emotional state was far from normal.

As that stage of grief dragged on I began seriously to think I needed help, outside, possibly professional, help. I felt trapped in my grief. I had difficulty sleeping and when I did sleep I had vivid nightmares about death. During the day I couldn't liberate my mind from thinking about Will. But the problem was where to look for help.

At that time, bereavement counselling had not become the established service now offered by a number of organizations. Compassionate Friends, the organization for bereaved parents, did exist, but no one told me about it until much later. Had I known about them, I am sure that talking with other bereaved parents would, at a particular stage of my grief, have helped me greatly. As a bereaved parent, you feel that no one else, except another bereaved parent, can in any way begin to understand your feelings. I felt that then and I feel it now.

For these reasons, I am not sure how I would have responded to the offer, had it been made, of professional bereavement counselling. However, I do know that I would have greatly appreciated some person – a professional or a fellow sufferer – saying to me, 'What you are feeling is OK. It is perfectly normal'.

The growth in the availability of bereavement counselling is one of the major changes that has happened since the death of Will. Its growth has been part of the movement to break down the taboos that had grown up earlier this century surrounding dying, death and bereavement. Geoffrey Gorer was one the first to draw attention to the British way of dying in the mid-twentieth century. In the early sixties, following a personal experience of bereavement, he made a study of the subject and wrote *Death, Grief and Mourning in Contemporary Britain*. He found that, 'Most people, it would seem, now die alone, except for medical attendants; less than a quarter of the bereaved were present when their relative died, and nearly two thirds of those present were women'. His picture of death in Britain in the sixties is cold, depersonalized and frightening. The most chilling line in the whole description is, 'Nearly all the children died in hospital, alone'. It is a shocking indictment of our society that we have become so frightened and alienated from dying and death that we allow children to die alone in hospital. My son died alone.

Will died in intensive care the day after he had had surgery. Thanks to the League of Friends, we had been given a room across the road from the hospital in which we could stay together during the period of Will's surgery. At least we had a private place to wait. The morning following his operation, we visited Will in intensive care and were allowed to see him briefly. We were then ushered away. They told us that they were worried about him and we were advised to return to our room and wait. We had one phone call to warn us that Will had had a cardiac arrest and that things did not look good.

> Soon after the phone rang again, again Ed answered. This time I saw him crumple, controlling his choking just long enough to hear the news. He didn't need to tell me. I knew Will was dead.

I was not with my child when he died. That is a source of deep, deep pain and loss to me. Perhaps I should have demanded to have been there and asserted our presence in the high-tech world of intensive care, but overawed and frightened, it is hard to be assertive. Afterwards, I wondered whether or not the doctors and nurses felt that the presence of the parents would inhibit their desperate final attempts to save Will's life. However, I expect the truth was that it just didn't enter their heads to ask us if we wanted to be present.

Sensitivity to the needs of parents has increased since the death of Will. It is slowly filtering through to hospital wards that, ultimately, in the fullness of time, it is less painful for the bereaved to have been there. This change of attitude has been influenced greatly by the hospice movement. Dame Cicely Saunders, who founded the movement, has always recognized that care of the dying is also care of the bereaved. In her view, dying alone should not happen unless the individual specifically wants to die alone. Respecting the rights of the dying is central to her philosophy. Respecting the emotional needs of those to be bereaved is also part of her philosophy. Excluding them would be anathema. Reverend Ian Ainsworth Smith, one of the new breed of full-time hospital chaplain's, spoke of how the ideas of the hospice movement had influenced him and others of his generation, including nurses, during their training. Through people like him, the philosophy has spread out and now influences the ways in which hospitals 'treat' death. How a death in a hospital is handled by the professionals, as I am only too painfully aware, can have a profound affect on the bereaved.

After we had been told of Will's death, we were asked if we wanted to see him. We said we did. The hospital staff were clearly upset, awkward and embarrassed about his death. He had been laid out in a small, glass-partitioned section of the unit and they had stuck brown paper on the windows. The sister stood over us as we sat by him. She was uncomfortable. We, even in that moment of brutal reality, were inhibited by her watchful eye. At least seeing Will dead was a crucial starting point in the slow process of accepting that he was dead. Years later, when I read that parents are now encouraged to stay with their children as long as they wish, to hold them, to feel the last warmth of their child leaving them, I ached to have been able to have held Will. To have felt that transition from life to death. It would have softened the brutality of his death.

Many years later, a close friend, Jill, died. She had cancer and spent the last two months of her life in a Marie Curie hospice, Edenhall. I had visited her regularly, both at home and after she had been admitted to Edenhall. My daughter, Jessie, was friends with Jill's two daughters and also knew Jill well. Jessie accompanied me, or her friends, on several visits and I know that she was glad that she had done so. There was a point when all of us who knew Jill felt that she, as the old phrase goes, had decided to 'turn her face to the wall'. After this point, it was not long before she died. As soon as I was told of her death, I went to see her children and her husband. From their house, directed by some strong inner urge, I drove up to Edenhall. I knew I wanted to see Jill and I wanted to do it alone. On arriving at Edenhall, a nurse greeted me. 'I've come to see Jill', I said. The nurse accompanied me to Jill's room and asked if I wanted anything. I said, 'No, thank you'. The nurse then withdrew. Some time later, she popped her head round the door and asked if I was all right and did I want a cup of tea. I replied that I was fine and she left.

My privacy was respected and yet there was, clearly, a watchful eye kept on me, just in case I needed someone. I deeply appreciated their respect and care for me.

In the peace and privacy of that room, I sat by Jill. She lay in bed, dressed in her nightie, no different from the time I had seen her two days before, except that the pain had gone from her face. She looked very young and, I know it sounds clichéd, but it was true, very peaceful. I sat and cried. Slowly, as my tears became more uncontrollable, I realized that my tears were not just for Jill. I was very sad that I had lost a close friend, but my tears were for something else. Wrenched to the surface were quite unexpected feelings, ones I was quite unprepared for – those of anger and pain. I sat there thinking, this is what I should have been allowed to do with Will. *This* is what was denied me. The hospital had not given us the opportunity to be with Will in privacy for as long as we wished. It was as though their embarrassment and their sense of failure, though I never felt that they had 'failed', overrided our emotional needs. When we visited Will, it was signalled very clearly to us that this 'viewing' was in their space to which we had been invited and, once there, we were to be watched over. Jill died in 1990, 15 years after Will's death. It took all that time and a particular experience to trigger my feelings of anger about a denied experience.

No one should be denied the chance to privately deal with the death of someone they love. Knowing how deeply the long-term effect had been on me of the treatment of us at Will's death, I asked Reverend Ainsworth Smith how the death of a child in a neonatal unit would be handled now. I asked, in particular, whether or not parents would be invited into the high-tech world to be with their child when death was imminent. He was somewhat taken aback by my question. His surprise at my question was not that I was asking if something totally impossible could happen, but that it was so much part of their practice now that he could not imagine parents being excluded if they requested to be present. Being present would not just be offered to parents, but they would be encouraged to be there. I commented on the marked change in attitude and practice that had occurred over the intervening years.

Reverend Ainsworth Smith stressed how central *nurses* had been in helping to bring about change. 'They have gained more confidence and responsibility', he said and added, 'And are much more able to act on their gut feelings'. Many nurses are themselves parents. Helping parents through the death of their child, which I am sure is painful and upsetting for the nurses, must also, ultimately, be more rewarding for the nursing staff than shutting the parents out.

After seeing Will, we saw the senior registrar; he said how sorry he was and we believed him. After that meeting, we left.

> So Ed and I walked out of the hospital dazed, shocked and fragile and the only help offered to us was 'just to go home'. I felt we were an embarrassment to them. Not just to Dr Y but to the whole system. Despite the fact that it is a situation with which they have to deal with quite frequently they had no training, no personnel, no organisation to deal with it. They are there to fight for life and when that life ends their role in relation to that life and those involved ends.

No one even asked how we might get home. Fortunately, my parents were on hand to pick up the pieces. I wondered whether or not such abandonment of parents by the hospital still happened or whether or not that, too, had changed. Reverend Ainsworth Smith stressed that he could not speak for other hospitals, but that there was a consensus of opinion throughout the medical profession about what was now regarded as good practice at such times. At St George's Hospital, where he works, those concerned have drawn up their own code of practice and he gave me a copy of it. Part of it deals with the formalities of death, particularly about 'notification'. This lays out very clearly what the duties are of the registrar on the day following the death of a child in the paediatric intensive care unit. The document stresses that these duties '*must be completed by the registrar immediately before undertaking other duties in the hospital*'. Notifying the social worker and the chaplain are one of the registrar's immediate duties. The procedure means that support should immediately be on hand for the bereaved should they need it. There is a longer list of 'notifications' that are to be made by other members of the team. The list includes 'Mother's obstetrician'. Reverend Ainsworth Smith explained that if the child had been born at St George's, he would personally get the file out and ensure that the information about its death was put in the mother's file. If born elsewhere, he would write and hope the information would be incorporated into the mother's file. It was, I thought, a touch of real sensitivity. There is nothing so distressful, I know, as attending an antenatal clinic and being cheerfully asked by the nurse, the doctor and others who look at one's file how your child is getting on. The list also includes notification of the GP and the health visitor. 'That flushes out the good ones from the bad', the Reverend commented. My health visitor visited me; my GP did not.

Greater recognition of the emotional needs of the bereaved by hospitals can make a great difference to how people begin the deal with their grief. Professional bereavement counsellors can and do help many people. In a society that still fears those who mourn and censures the expression of grief, there is little collective social knowledge of how to support people. Professionals can help, though, unfortunately, with recognition of bereavement come new standards of human behaviour. In campaigning to allow people to express their grief and not be socially pressured to hide it, a new pressure has emerged – the pressure to grieve 'well'. In all the very important campaigns to recognize and humanize birth, death and grief, there has been a down side – each has set new standards of human behaviour. Women who do not give birth naturally often feel failures. The 'good death', having been out of vogue for at least a century, is back on the list of human achievements, an achievement for which one can only win a posthumous award. The person who 'successfully' bereaves is one who comes through grieving to a state of acceptance and equanimity. They can count themselves as one of life's achievers.

When I wrote *Will, My Son*, I thought that I had come 'successfully' through my grief to such a state of acceptance and equanimity. I felt no embarrassment then writing about the stages of grief I had gone through. I was campaigning for recognition of grief and that grieving is not contained within a matter of weeks, months or even a year or two. Many think getting through the first year is the major hurdle. They are then deeply distressed to find the second year even harder. For me, I thought the lifting of the clouds would come with the birth of Jessie. Immediately after her birth I was high – 'high from relief, ecstasy and the energy gained from the life force of birth' – but I was totally unprepared, emotionally, for what was to hit me when I got home with her.

> To hold a baby again, to change its nappies, to feed it and play with it just made me re-live doing all those things with Will. It made me confront all I had been evading since his death. No one had warned me such feelings are common following the birth of a second child when the first has died. I felt guilty that I was mourning Will when I had Jessie and because of my guilt I could not talk about the fact that I was going through a second period of mourning for which I had been totally unprepared.
>
>   . . .
>
>   My problem in relating to Jessie and in coming to terms with the fact she was not Will were solved more by Jessie than me. As she developed and grew, asserting herself as a very definite individual, I compared her less and less to Will and began to relate to her as Jessie. I mourned less and less for Will and became more and more involved with Jessie. I had loved her from birth, but I had to develop a love for her as Jessie not as an image of someone I had lost.

Having come through this second period of mourning, I believed that there was a time frame and my time of grieving was through. I confidently wrote in *Will, My Son*

> With her [Jessie's] help, with Ed's love and support and with the support of so many other friends and relatives, particularly my parents, I now feel I have come through.

I now know that when I wrote this I had merely 'come through' a *stage* of grief. I had not, as I thought and no doubt the reader thought, come through grieving altogether. I realize that, in making such an assertion, I, like others, have contributed to an assumption that there is a time frame to grief.

The act of going public, of publishing under one's own name is itself a sign of having not just survived but, at some level, come to terms with the experience. Like me, most people who write of their grief seem to write at a particular stage. It is at this stage that one feels one has come through: the point when one feels that one has reached some kind of emotional normality, when one can function socially and at work and when one has found some kind of acceptance of the reality of the death. Because of the confidence gained from having survived this stage, one feels able to speak out.

To help him come to terms with his grief following the sudden death of his 11-year-old elder son, Jonathan, Christopher Leach wrote *Letter To A Younger Son*. It is a moving and eloquent exploration, covering the first year of his grief. The book ends as the first anniversary of Jonathan's death approaches. Approaching this anniversary, Christopher Leach wrote in *Letter To A Younger Son* three sections entitled 'What I have discovered?', 'What I have learned?' and 'What do I believe?' His answers to his own questions reveal that he discovered and learned much and found a firm belief. He discovered much about the pain of grief and that 'tragedy need not diminish those who suffer it'. He found that his belief in life 'is strengthened by death'. His section on 'What I have learned?' is an eloquent testimony to the way in which the experience of 'a deeper grief than I thought possible' can not only be survived, but can cause profound change. Christopher Leach learned 'what is important; that faced with the ultimate, things move to a correct proportion'. In this process of learning, meaning also returned to his life. The person who had contemplated suicide in the dark days after Jonathan's death could write a year later: 'I have been granted a certain time to walk about this Earth, and to take a look at its marvels and its follies – and perhaps contribute to both – and what I do matters'.

Christopher Leach goes on to write, 'Being human, I am still hurt. Being human I am not reconciled; yet part of me soars'. It is the final phrase that we cling to. It is the message contained in this phrase, informed by what we have read earlier in the book, that we take away with us. Those who are not bereaved – who fear that they, too, may one day have to face such savage pain – want to know not only that you can survive, but that inner strength and greater understanding may be gained. The dust jacket of *A Letter To A Younger Son* tells the reader that Christopher Leach 'rises from the ashes of heartbreak and anger to a personal affirmation that offers strength and solace to anyone who must suffer such loss'. Indeed, when I read the book in 1982 (it was published in paperback a year after *Will, My Son*), I indeed took strength and solace from it. I came away from reading it holding on to those things Christopher Leach had learned and discovered and to the phrase, 'but part of me soars'. I identified with what he wrote. As a survivor, I also identified with and understood his need to affirm the positive. In the final paragraph of *Will, My Son*, I wrote:

> But time and events have stopped me running away from his death. Now I run because like Dr Sassall interviewed by John Berger in *A Fortunate Man*, 'Whenever I am reminded of death . . . I think of my own and this makes me try to work harder'. Such running is an affirmation, not an evasion, of life and in my case an affirmation of the preciousness of time and love. That is Will's legacy.

Just as I am sure that Christopher Leach would say his statement still holds true for him today, so does mine. Will's legacy lives with me and I will take it to my grave. At the base line, I know what is important. Sometimes the base line recedes from my vision, but I always return to it. The knowledge of what is important to me puts all the other problems of life in perspective. There are times when I have been depressed, when things in my life are going badly and, sooner or later in my spiral downwards of self-pity, I will say to myself, 'Come on, stop. These aren't bad times; you *know* what bad times really are'. This knowledge is strength, a strength that does not diminish or become diluted with the years. Affirming what I have gained from bereavement is not just an attempt to convince myself and the world that I have salvaged something from death. It is what I profoundly feel.

However, bringing this affirmation into the foreground like

this is to give the impression that this is the *only* long-term legacy. We all, for our own reasons, want to believe that the nightmare can be put behind and that we can come through. We can then go forward. It is as though we are Hollywood movie makers, wanting to give the world a happy ending. The classic fictional exploration of grief, Frances Hodgson Burnett's *The Secret Garden*, does just this. The story is about a young, orphaned girl, Mary, who is sent back from India to live with her uncle, Mr Craven and his invalid son, Colin in Yorkshire. The secret garden of the title is the place where Mr Craven's wife had been killed by a branch falling on her. After the accident, Mr Craven locked up the walled garden and threw away the key. Ten years later, Mary finds the key, unlocks the garden and, with time, unlocks the father and son who are trapped in grief and the repercussions of this grief. Colin slowly becomes normal and healthy, able to walk and run. Mr Craven, one day, finds the garden unlocked and goes in. In this action he confronts his grief and, in so doing, finds a future. He embraces his son Colin and, instead of selling the house and garden in Yorkshire, which he had been planning to do, agrees that they should all stay there. The book ends with them all beginning to rebuild their lives. The message of the book is that grief has to be confronted and that, if you can confront it, you can move forward and live and love again. While in no way wishing to undercut the central message of the story, the 'happily ever after' ending is another example of the wish to highlight only the positive. In effect, it is saying you can achieve 'personal growth' (a phrase much used by the professionals) by dealing with your grief and, having dealt with it and grown as a person, then your grieving will be a thing of the past. The two are not exclusive, however. In my experience, I have found greater self-understanding *at the same time* as living with an ever-present grief.

The difference in the feelings I had when writing this book compared to those I had when writing *Will, My Son* is that I now feel deeply embarrassed to admit to my grief. There are two sources of this embarrassment. How can I, I ask myself, be making such a fuss when others have suffered much greater losses. I watch the television coverage of Yugoslavia - mothers who have lost one, two or even more children, fathers who have lost their wives and whole families, grandparents who would have laid down their own lives if this had meant that they would have ensured that their children and their children's children could have survived them. I watch scenes from Africa - families decimated, a mother crouched over the dead body of her child. My loss is just one, personal loss. I should, I argue to myself, put my own experience into some kind of wider perspective. In so doing, I should be able to, maybe not forget, but at least put the experience well behind me and move on.

My other fear is that if I admit to still grieving people will immediately think I need professional help and advise me to have either professional counselling, therapy or analysis. The new pressure to successfully grieve has left me feeling a failure. This feeling of failure is not helped by reading literature by professionals who all talk about working through to resolution. Judy Tatelbaum, an American, perhaps best sums up this expectation by calling a chapter in her book *The Courage to Grieve* [Lippincott and Crowell 1980] 'Finishing'. She writes 'How do we know when we are finished?', and goes on to say, 'We are finished when our grief feelings seem dissipated, when we can think of the loss or the loved one without pain . . .' On this latter point alone I rate 'unfinished'.

In the course of writing this book I was made aware that I have clearly not finished on another count, too. Judy Tatelbaum advises, 'dreams can be signals of our unfinished business'. After writing the first draft, I went through a week of nights disturbed by vivid nightmares. I had not had these particular nightmares since the year following the death of Will. There is obviously, then, unfinished business in my unconscious. It does not surprise me. I defy any parent who has experienced the death of a child not to, at times, throughout the rest of their lives think of their dead child with pain or to have in their unconscious scars left by that pain. This seems to me to be normal. Trying, however, to cling on to what one thinks is normality against a tide of belief that emotional business can and should be finished is hard. In denying the ongoing pain and in talking about what one can learn and gain from grief, a certain process of beatification happens.

'They that mourn', as St Matthew claimed are, 'Blessed'. Grief becomes ennobled and ennobling. It *is* or can be, if not ennobling, enriching, but to speak only of this is to omit the dark side. It is a dishonesty and one that belies the reality of the experience, or at least my reality.

One of the problems with trying to explore the long-term effects of grief, of whether I am normal or abnormal, is that so few have written about it - or, rather, many, I believe, have written in one way or another about their feelings, but few have gone public with them. C. S. Lewis clearly felt to go public with his feelings of grief following the death of his wife was impossible. His classic, *A Grief Observed* was first published in 1961 under a pseudonym, the author's identity only being revealed after his death in 1963. Sean O'Casey kept a secret diary of his grief for four years following the death of his son Niall. His wife Eileen only found it after O'Casey's death. It is a reflection of our society this century that two major writers, who could explore in public a whole range of other feelings, could not speak of their own deepest feelings.

Perhaps, though, it is only by writing in secret that the savagery of the pain can be expressed. The first entry of O'Casey's diary states that on 30 December 1956, 'Niall died'. The second entry is for the 13 April 1957: 'Oh, God, to think of it; I buried a father when I was a little boy, and a son when I was an old, old man'. Four years later, O'Casey had found no resolution, or finishing, of his grief. On 31 December, 1960, he wrote, 'These weekly tributes to him are trifling and useless, bringing him no nearer, nor easing the ache of the sorrow of his going. I thought they might, but still each day he comes to mind; and always will till I go too'. On reading *A Grief Observed* you are left knowing that all is not resolved. C. S. Lewis writes, 'For in grief nothing "stays put"', and he goes on to ask, 'How often - will it be for always? - how often will the vast emptiness astonish me like a complete novelty and make me say, "I never realised my loss till this moment"? The same leg is cut off time and time again. The first plunge of the knife into the flesh is felt again and again'.

I cannot give a specific number in reply to the question 'How often?', but, 18 years later, I know that, from time to time, the pain of that first plunge can suddenly, from somewhere deep inside me, surface. Before I was bereaved I had assumed that grief, like a photograph, would slowly fade with time. I have learned otherwise. Somewhere inside is an album of pristine prints, as sharp and as clear as the day these images were imprinted on me. I have learned to live with this. There are moments when I can summon up these images in calm, but they can still flash up unexpectedly and painfully.

C. S Lewis and Sean O'Casey provide a vivid insight into the anguish and pain of grief and of their failure to find any permanent resolution, but the period of their lives that they write about is, in physical time, relatively brief. It is very hard to find out, to even glimpse, how people live through the rest of their lives with grief. Once that first stage of grief, which people have spoken and written about, has been passed through, a silence descends. In the absence of the bereaved writing about how grief has affected their lives, I have looked to other possible sources of information.

Biographers, probing people's lives, might, I thought, provide insight. I should have realized that biographers are as wary of probing the ravages of grief as anyone else. At university in the sixties, I did a thesis on Sean O'Casey for my MA. It was my first real exposure to biographies. It struck me even then in my youth and innocence that what I felt had to be a profoundly important experience in someone's life was ignored by those who claimed to be writing about the man, his life and work. One biographer, David Krause, had seen it only necessary to register in a footnote that O'Casey's son, Niall, 'died suddenly of leukemia in 1956'. In another study by Saros Cowasjee entitled *Sean O'Casey: The man behind the plays*, the death of Niall is not even mentioned, although mention is made of his other son and daughter. As O'Casey's own autobiography (a sequence of six volumes) was written and published before his son's death, I was left with little detail of this major event in his life. It was only with the publication of *Sean* [Macmillan 1971] in 1971, a biography written about O'Casey by his wife, Eileen, that I not only learned of the circumstances of Niall's death, but the devastation it had wreaked on the family. Eileen attempted suicide but, after that attempt, she wrote, 'We both knew it was essential to carry on living instead of indulging in selfish grief. Sean threw himself into his work; I went on with my everyday life, and we got over the time somehow, as one must'. It was only in 1991 that the depth of Sean O'Casey's grief was revealed through the publication of his diary.

Since the death of Will, whenever I am reading a biography and the subject has experienced the death of a child, I immediately look for some further illumination or exploration of the effect this experience had on the subject's life. Time and time again, I am disappointed. For example, I read Jill Benton's biography of Naomi Mitchison. Suddenly, in the middle of love affairs, work and defending her brother Jack against a charge brought against him by Cambridge University for 'gross habitual immorality', Jill Benton writes, 'Willing as Naomi was to take on life – in her loving, in her writing, in her philosophy – it was death that shook her to the depths of her being. In 1927, her oldest child, nine-year-old Geoff, died of spinal meningitis'. Not only did her son die, but Naomi Mitchison's brother, to whom she had been close, blamed *her* for Geoff's death. Naomi, thus, not only lost her son, but, when she most needed the support of her brother, she was rejected by him. It takes only three short paragraphs for the author to deal with this chapter in the life of Naomi Mitchison. Most contemporary biographers, like Jill Benton, unlike those writing about O'Casey in the sixties can, at least, bring themselves to mention the subject of death, but, invariably, it is quickly left, with some such phrase as, 'it profoundly affected the rest of his/her life'.

This phrase and its variations, such as she/he never got over it', I am familiar with. More than one friend has told me that their mother suffered a bereavement. One, I remember, said that her mother had lost a baby at birth, or shortly after birth, and then added, 'She has never forgotten it'. Reverend Ainsworth Smith told me of an experience he had had when visiting, an old lady nearing the end of her life on one of the wards. He asked her, 'How many children have you?' She replied, 'Five', hesitated and then said, 'No, six.' In tears, she then told Reverend Ainsworth Smith of her 'sixth child' – a baby who had died at birth or soon after birth. 'Fifty years later, she still remembered the child vividly and cried'. Reverend Ainsworth Smith said this to me, knowing I was looking for reassurance. I *am* reassured to know that others, like me, do not forget, but I want to know more. I want to know how it affected them and in what ways.

A rare insight into this legacy came through reading J. G. Ballard's autobiography, *The Kindness of Women* [Grafton, 1992]. It is a sequel to the *Empire Of The Sun*, which had dealt with his childhood years in a Japanese civilian prisoner of war camp in China. *The Kindness Of Women* is about his life as an adult in Britain. Central to the story is the death of his wife and the emotional legacy of this bereavement. If you read the blurb, and this was written in 1991, you would not know that his wife had died, only that 'his world was ripped apart by family tragedy' and, following this tragedy, 'He plunges into the maelstrom of the 1960s, an instigator and subject of every aspect of cultural, social and sexual experimentation'. In the middle of this maelstrom, another thing the blurb does not mention is that J. G. Ballard chose, against the prevailing social attitudes of the time, which thought fathers incapable of such a thing, to bring up his children on his own. It is, in many ways, a very powerful and well-written book. To me its particular power lies in the fact that J. G. Ballard, almost 30 years after the death of his wife, had felt it important to not only recount her death, but to explore how her death (and the experiences of his childhood) had affected and influenced his life.

When I say that I still grieve, I do not want to give the impression that I go around in a state of grieving. I do not literally, or metaphorically, go around in mourning dress. In my daily life, I do not consciously carry my grief with me most of the time. However, the person I am who goes around has been remoulded by grief. When Will died, part of me died. In the novel *Indigo* [Vintage, 1992], Marina Warner, in describing the effect of the death of a daughter on the main character, Sycorax, wrote, 'Her daughter became a ghost limb that aches at night and sets the whole body burning with its absence'. Marina Warner then, through the thoughts of Sycorax, speaks further of the physicality of her loss: 'No men ever feel such pain for their offspring, she thought, no matter how much they try to merge with their wives, even when they gash themselves in imitation of menarche, and pretend to struggle in the coils of labour alongside them during the birth, no matter how much they love the child. It originates in flesh . . .' I cannot speak for the pain of men. The loss of someone you love causes deep pain for all human beings – as Christopher Leach, Sean O'Casey and other men will testify to – but, for mothers, there is a physicality in this loss and it does originate in the flesh. Will was part of my body, part of the physical oneness that is the mother–child relationship.

With the rare exception, I can only assume that other people – for I do not believe that I am unique – sense that a time comes when one should be silent about one's grief. Phillippe Aries wrote in *The Hour Of Our Death*, 'The pain of loss may continue to exist in the secret heart of the survivor, but the rule today, almost throughout the West, is that he must never show it'. This statement is, I have found, to be true not just of the first stages of grief, but of the ongoing experience. To all intents and purposes, in public, one has to pretend that it is an experience one never had because to claim it in any way is to cross the line of accepted behaviour.

For all the books that have been written over the past two or three decades calling for a recognition of grief, for all the television programmes (of which I have made one) legitimizing the expressions of grief, for all the development of professional help and counselling for the bereaved, little has actually changed in social attitudes. To show or even to mention in public that one has been bereaved is still taboo. The bereaved, particularly parents who have lost a child, will recount how people literally cross the street rather than have to deal with acknowledging them and their loss. People *continue* to literally, and in their social behaviour, cross the street.

Over the years I have noticed no discernible change in people's ability to deal with my answer to their question, 'How many children do you have?' I know the question is asked in innocence, the questioner having no prior knowledge of the pain contained in the answer. I refuse to deny the existence of Will. I refuse to pretend that he never existed and so I answer 'Two, but my first died'. There is a silence. The questioner then usually mumbles an embarrassed, 'I'm sorry'. I then feel responsible for having caused such embarrassment and quickly talk on about Jessie and how she is growing up and is fine and healthy, then move the subject on. There are one or two variations to this scenario. One is that, after saying 'I'm sorry', a further question is asked, 'How long ago?' When my reply indicates that it was some years ago, at least more than two or three, there is visible relief on the person's face, sometimes expressed in some such phrase as, 'Oh well, that's some time ago now'. It is as if they are saying, 'That's OK. It is passed'. Another twist is if I give my full answer and say, 'Two, but my first died. He was a Down's Syndrome baby and died following open heart surgery'. In the interests of my own self-protection, I rarely give this answer because I know that, all too frequently, the answer will be, 'It was probably for the best'. Very occasionally, a person replies to my normal answer with a direct question like, 'How did he die?', or, 'How old was he?' Almost certainly this questioner has experienced the death of someone they have loved. Sometimes the person replies directly with this information. In these situations, we both feel the sudden relief of speaking the same emotional language. Relief at the safety of being able to talk of an experience without continually assessing the feelings of the other.

My experience of the death of my child is an experience that informs my thoughts, feelings and attitudes. It is, however, an experience that I only occasionally own up to in any public forum, whether this be at work, at a dinner party or any other public situation. I cannot use my experience to explain myself, my thoughts or my feelings. The rare occasions when I have done so have triggered such acute embarrassment and awkwardness for the receivers of this information that the conversation is stopped in its tracks, then quickly changed. To bring my experience up in an argument, I am aware, is looked upon as not playing by the Queensberry Rules. It is received as a below-the-belt hit and, therefore, should not have been made. It is ruled out of order. I was having dinner with friends once and, at one point, the discussion turned to the case - then being argued in the courts and in the media - of a young man left brain dead following the Hillsborough disaster. The debate centred on the ethics of turning off his life support systems. After joining in the discussion at an emotional distance, I then introduced another level to the debate. I made a comment about the complexity of the issue and the difficulty others have in understanding the feelings of those involved in such a decision. 'I know', I said, 'I've been there. We were given the option of leaving Will to die'. I could feel the knife cut through the air surrounding the dinner table. I knew I had gone too far and had crossed a line. The conversation was quickly returned to emotional safety.

In general, it is men who most rigidly adhere to the emotional Queensberry Rules of debate. Women are more tolerant because, for them, emotional experiences have always been part of what they regard and accept as knowledge. They accept as evidence personal life experiences and offer their own as support. They form much of the fabric of women's conversations and relationships. However, I have found, even with some women, that my experience of bereavement is too savage and unnerving to be allowed into this human exchange.

The denial of my experience takes another form, too. From time to time, I will find myself in a discussion on some topic that relates to my experiences. Even though the other people in the group, or even some of them, will know my story, they will never invite me to contribute my thoughts and feelings, based on my experience. If I had been divorced, suffered a serious illness, had had a miscarriage or experienced any number of other traumatic experiences, these would be recognized. Because Will died, the denial is not only of his death but also of his disability. Any understanding of Down's Syndrome, the condition, the feelings of parents, the ethical issues, the attitudes of the medical profession or society in general, I am not expected to have or to express.

It is not everyone who denies my experience, though. There are those who lived with me through the experience and recognize that it does inform my thoughts and feelings. A few others have taken on board this part of my past and recognize it. For instance, I could not have made the documentary series *Merely Mortal* for Channel 4 in the mid-eighties had not my colleague Rachael Trezise accepted, with great understanding, my experience as part of the knowledge that informed the series. However, the vast majority, particularly those who have not suffered the loss of someone they have closely loved, deny it. In this denial, an extraordinary reversal of human behaviour happens. If someone is hurt, then normal human behaviour is for others to tend and comfort them, to care for them and their needs. However, if one is hurting as a result of grief, it is the bereaved who have to learn, very quickly, to be considerate of *other* people's emotions. They quickly learn that they, as mourners, create fear in others. Their presence touches on people's deepest fears and they learn that no one wants a mourner in their midst. Contrary to St Matthew's exhortation, 'Blessed are they that mourn; for they shall be comforted', it is more a case of, 'Cursed are they that mourn; for they are like unto the shadow of death'. Quickly, as a mourner, you learn to hide the pain to protect others. There is a long way to go and a major change in social attitudes is required before the bereaved will be able to 'come out'.

In *Will, My Son* I wrote:

> I still want to talk about him not so much because I any longer have
> a need but because to be silent about him is to deny his existence.

I do still talk about him because I refuse to deny his existence, but, also, I have learned over the years that I have a *need* to talk about him. It is not the raw, immediate need of the early days that I realized, when writing the above, I had passed through. It is the need to affirm it as part of my life's experience. Although the death of a child in the West, outside of wars, in now, thankfully, uncommon, we all, at some time in our lives, will experience the loss of someone we love and care for. In denying others the right to claim their experience, each person will find that they are denying themselves this right when their time comes. They are condemning themselves to, one day, carrying their pain and their history secretly.

In denying grief, we are, in fact, denying death. For, more than anything, what grief does is remind us of our mortality. In 1987,

I wrote in *Merely Mortal* (the book that accompanied the Channel 4 television series of the same name):

> We do shrink from the knowledge of death, preferring to cruise through life in the implicit assumption that we are immortal until suddenly the death of someone we love brings us up with a sharp jolt. Our confidence in the certainties of life are shattered. Despite the fact that we are aware of others dying in wars, in famines, in accidents, in cancer or geriatric wards, we do not relate those deaths to ourselves. It is only when someone we love dies that we realise that others we love can also die - most of all that we ourselves can die. That realisation of mortality is a realisation of what it is to be human.

What I did not write then was that it is Will to whom I am indebted for this realization. This is Will's legacy.

Further reading

DISABILITY

There is now a wide range of books available on many aspects of Down's Syndrome - medical, developmental, social and legal. The following are books or pamphlets that I have found interesting.

E. Byrne, C.C. Cunningham and P. Sloper, *Families And Their Children with Down's Syndrome* (Routledge Chapman & Hall, 1988)
Cliff Cunningham, *Down's Syndrome* (Souvenir Press, 1990)
C.F. Goodey (Ed.), *Living In The Real World: Families speak about Down's Syndrome* (Twenty-One Press, 1991)
Sheila Jupp, *Making The Right Start* (Opened Eye Publications, 1992)
John O'Brien and Alan Tyne, *The Principle of Normalization: A foundation for effective services* (Values Into Action, 1981)
Hazel Morgan, *Through Peter's Eyes* (Arthur James Ltd, 1990)
Ann Shearer, *Everybody's Ethics: What future for handicapped babies?* (Values Into Action, 1984)
Brian Stratford, *Down's Syndrome: Past, Present and Future* (Penguin, 1989)
Alison Wertheimer, *According to the Papers: Press reporting on people with learning difficulties* (Values Into Action, 1988)
Wolf Wolfensberger, *A Brief Introduction to Social Role Valorization as a High-order Concept for Restructuring Human Services* (Syracuse University Press, 1992)

GRIEF

Philippe Aries, *The Hour Of Our Death* (Penguin Books, 1983)
Philippe Aries, *Western Attitudes Toward Death* (John Hopkins Press, 1983)
Sarah Boston and Rachael Trezise, *Merely Mortal: Coping with Dying, Death and Bereavement* (Methuen, 1987)
Geoffrey Gorer, *Death, Grief and Mourning in Contemporary Britain* (Crescent Press, 1965)
Christopher Leach, *Letter to a Younger Son* (Arrow Books, 1981)
C.S. Lewis, *A Grief Observed* (Faber and Faber, 1978)
Sean O'Casey, *Niall* (Calder Publications Limited, 1991)

Useful addresses

DISABILITY

The Centre for Studies on
   Integration in Education
4th Floor
415 Edgware Road
London NW2 6NB
Tel: 081-452 8642

Down's Syndrome Association
155 Mitchum Road
London SW17 9PG
Tel: 081-682 4001

IPSEA (Independent Panel for
   Special Education Advice)
c/o John Wright
12 Marsh Road
Tillingham
Essex CM0 7SZ
Tel: 0621 779781

Mencap (Royal Society for Mentally
   Handicapped Children and
   Adults)
133 Golden Lane
London EC1Y 0RT
Tel: 071-454 0454

The Portsmouth Down's Syndrome
   Trust
Psychology Department
Portsmouth Polytechnic
King Charles Street
Portsmouth PO1 2ER

Values Into Action
Oxford House
Derbyshire Street
London E2 6HG
Tel: 071-729 5436

GRIEF

There is a variety of local and
national services for the bereaved.
The following are national
organizations that give information
on local services and on
organizations offering advice and
help for specific needs.

National Association of
   Beareavement Services
20 Norton Folgate
London E1 6DB
Tel: 071-247 1081

Cruse
The National Organization for the
   Widowed and their Children
126 Sheen Road
Richmond
Surrey TW9 1UR
Tel: 081-940 4818

Compassionate Friends
53 North Street
Bristol BS3 1EN
Tel: 0272 539634

(Compassionate Friends offers a
support service for bereaved parents.)